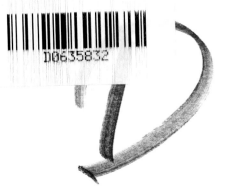

The Ultimate Guide to WEIGHT TRAINING for BASEBALL and SOFTBALL

third edition

Prior to beginning any exercise program, you must consult with your physician.
You must also consult your physician before increasing the intensity of your training.

Any application of the recommended material in this book is at the sole risk of the reader, and at the reader's discretion. Responsibility of any injuries or other negative effects resulting from the application of any of the information provided within this book is expressly disclaimed.

Published by Price World Enterprises
5815 Landerbrook Drive
P.O. Box 24434
Cleveland, OH 44124

Book design and layout by Alexandru Dan Georgescu
Book design by Jeff Ross
Cover design by Alexandru Dan Georgescu
Interior photographs by Marc Gollub
Editing by Barb Greenberg
Editing and proofreading by Maryanne Haselow-Dulin

First edition: January 2003
ISBN: 1-932549-33-1

Printed in the United States of America

10 9 8 7 6 5 4 3 2 1

Special thanks to:
Dr. Marc B. Price CPFT for your expert insight and helpful contributions
Zack, David, and Gail Price for your support and encouragement to make this book possible.

The Ultimate Guide to WEIGHT TRAINING for BASEBALL and SOFTBALL

third edition

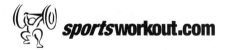

CONTENTS

Part I
BASEBALL/SOFTBALL SPECIFIC PROGRAM

Introduction

Both baseball and softball are sports where your overall level of strength and fitness is crucial to performing at the best of your abilities. Both sports require strength, power, speed, quickness, agility, flexibility, balance, muscular endurance, and stamina— each of which can be enhanced through a proper baseball- and softball-specific weight-training program. This book focuses on how to develop your body in every area that is

> If you have any questions regarding sports weight training, please email trainer@sportsworkout.com.

most important to these sports. It also provides you with daily baseball- and softball-specific programs designed for the off-season, preseason, and in-season to maximize your playing potential.

With the exception of a few minor details, the sports of baseball and softball are virtually identical. Both involve batting, pitching, fielding, and running. The only real differences between the two are the size of the ball and the release point of the pitcher. Weight training to improve your athletic potential for these sports is one and the same. Identical muscle groups, joints, and tendons are used while playing these sports, which is why this book focuses on the best ways to improve these vital areas. This book also provides you with an in-depth explanation of the theory behind every training technique to ensure you know exactly why you are doing what you are doing.

There are two requirements needed to be a good baseball and softball player: baseball- and softball-specific skills and proper conditioning. An important note must be made clear. Weight training will not directly improve your baseball and softball skills. However, it will make your entire body stronger and more powerful, which will give you greater bat and arm speed. It will also decrease your vulnerability to injury and increase your muscular endurance. All of these factors will increase your baseball and softball playing potential. If you train properly for baseball and softball, you will experience all of these benefits without sacrificing your technique on the field. In fact, proper weight training can enhance your technique by improving your flexibility and increasing your range of motion. This book not only contains a year-round baseball/softball-specific training program, but also includes over 50 additional 4-week programs so you can find exactly what you need.

Improper Training   Training improperly increases the risk of an injury occurring, and it can also set you further away from your goals. The goal of strength training for baseball and softball is not to build stiff, bulky muscles; it is to improve your game by increasing your speed, quickness, power, flexibility, muscular endurance, and balance. You want to build your muscles and improve flexibility in areas that are important to improving your performance on the diamond.

Major Benefits from Weight Training   Weight training for any sport provides you with two general benefits. It helps enhance your athletic performance and it helps reduce or prevent injury. Weight training also plays a major role in injury rehabilitation. Muscles that are well trained have been shown to recover faster from injuries, which will reduce chronic pain. Baseball and softball are outdoor sports and players are at the mercy of Mother Nature, who can be very unpleasant in the spring. Unfortunately, cold and wet weather elevate the risk of many injuries, including sprains and pulled muscles. With stronger muscles supporting your bones, tendons, and ligaments, you will be much less injury prone in all aspects of your life.

Common Baseball and Softball Injuries   The most common injuries experienced by baseball and softball players are in the shoulder and elbow. These injuries negatively affect throwing, fielding, and swinging, which necessitates taking injury-reducing precautions. Always stretch before lifting and playing, and weight train properly. The programs provided in this book are designed to train these and other areas of your body, minimizing your chances of getting injured. The programs strengthen both the internal and external rotators of your rotator cuffs to help maintain an injury-free shoulder. The programs also require performing both arm-extending (triceps) exercises and arm-contracting (biceps) exercises through their entire range of motion during the same training session, thus reducing the chances of elbow injuries by increasing both the strength and flexibility in your elbow joint.

Knee injuries and hamstring pulls are also very common among baseball and softball players. They can occur in many activities, including sliding, running, and diving. Similar to strengthening the elbow, training the muscles surrounding the knee is a good way to protect yourself from these injuries. Performing both leg-extending (thighs) and leg-contracting (hamstring) exercises on the same day through their entire range of motion both strengthens and increases the flexibility in the knee and hamstring.

Practice Makes Perfect While weight training for baseball and softball, it is crucial to continue practicing your skills. Your neurotransmitters will need to adapt to your newfound strength so you can convert it into power on the diamond. As important as strength and power are, they are not as important as technique. You need to be throwing the ball continuously and practicing your fielding and batting. Practice your throwing on the off days from the gym. Take grounders, go the batting cages, do some long and short throwing, and practice, practice, practice throughout the off-season.

Quickness vs. Speed The programs provided in this book are designed to enhance both your speed and your quickness, placing more emphasis on quickness. During the course of a game, quickness and acceleration are more important than overall speed. The longest runs made during the course of a game last no more than a few seconds: stealing a base, flagging down a fly, beating out an infield hit, stretching a double into a triple, and so forth. Infielders need to be able to get to balls hit up the middle or on the corners, and catchers need to explode out of the crouch to gun out a runner at second. By following the programs provided, you will increase your quickness and reduce your base path time.

Vital Body Parts

Throwing a baseball or softball and swinging a bat may not seem complex, but they are both multifaceted processes that involve muscles and joints from all parts of the body. Performing these activities as hard as your potential allows requires perfect technique and a maximum of strength, flexibility, and power. The most vital areas of the body for baseball and softball are the calves, thighs, hips, mid-section, lats, shoulders, and wrists. By improving aspects of one of these areas, you will improve your performance. By improving all of them, you will experience the benefits of weight training for baseball and softball. This book has you training most of the muscles of your body, with special emphasis on the areas listed above.

Calves

Throwing: The source of your throwing power comes from the lower body, initiating in the calves. The process of throwing begins when your toes push against the ground. The calves supply this initial "push," and the stronger they are, the better.

Running: The calves are the main source for the body's quickness and agility. Well-trained calves lead to faster acceleration and quicker side-to-side movements.

Exercises: Calf raises and seated calf raises.

Thighs and Hips

Throwing: Your throw gains a substantial amount of power from the thighs and hips. Just as you are about to release the ball, the back leg bends at the knee, which supplies power and momentum from the thighs and hips. The hips also help initiate the twisting motion in your body during a throw. Your total arm speed will benefit as the range of motion increases in the hips.

Batting: Batting also requires a major twist in the torso. Increased range of motion in the hips will help you get more leverage, which will lead to a more graceful, smooth, and explosive swing.

Running: Strong thighs and hips propel you to faster speeds, which can be beneficial when you need to bowl over a catcher who is in your path.

Exercises: Squats, lunges, leg extensions, etc.

A Note to Catchers: Be sure to perform squats with added emphasis. For every repetition, imagine yourself exploding out of the crouch to throw a runner out. The squat is the single most important weight-training exercise for you. It will develop your explosiveness and strength and, if done properly, will reduce knee injuries by strengthening your legs.

Mid-section

Throwing and swinging: The mid-section is where the lower body power gets transferred to the upper body and vice versa. Without a strong mid-section, you would be unable to apply your lower body explosion in your throws and swings. The speed at which your body rotates and twists during both your throws and swings comes from your mid-section. A strong mid-section is also a major contributor to balance and helps minimize shoulder and elbow trauma suffered from repeated throwing. Also, it takes less effort to check your swings with a well-trained mid-section. For the purposes of this manual, your mid-section is defined as the abdominals, lower back, and obliques.

Exercises: Any of a variety of abdominal, oblique, and lower back exercises can be performed, all of which can be found in this book.

Lats (Back) and Shoulders

Throwing: Your lats supply your shoulders with power, and it is your shoulders that enable you to throw the ball. Many areas of the shoulder are responsible for throwing, and each must be trained with equal consideration for purposes of muscle balance and arm acceleration and deceleration. The external rotators, front deltoids, and side deltoids are responsible for arm acceleration, and the rear deltoids and internal rotators are responsible for the deceleration of your arm.

Batting: The shoulders and lats supply you with the last major power surge during your swing. The stronger they are, the faster you can swing and the farther your balls will travel.

Fielding: While shoulders are often a forgotten part of fielding, they are of substantial importance. The ability to quickly take the ball out of your glove comes from your shoulders. A slow glove exchange can make the difference between a runner's being safe or out.

Hands and Wrists

Batting and Throwing: The hands are the final transfer point of power from your body to the bat, and they are the release point of the ball when throwing. Strong hands and wrists lead to better bat control, which can lead to opposite field homeruns and base hits off tough pitches. Strong hands and wrists also help pitchers throw different pitches and help reduce injuries that are caused from excessive curveballs.

Exercises: Forearm curls, wrist rollers, and hand grippers. Wrist rollers are the most effective because they strengthen both your forearm flexor and extensor muscles through their entire range of motion.

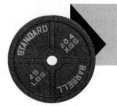
You can find the most effective wrist rollers on the market for a low price at www.sportsworkout.com

The Importance of Balance

Balance is essential in baseball and softball. If you are even slightly off balance, your swing will be off, your fielding will be off, and your game will suffer. There are two keys to achieving great body balance.

Train both sides of the body equally: It is critical that you train both sides of your body with equal frequency and intensity to achieve good balance. Training one side of the body more often or with greater intensity than the other can lead to one side being heavier than the other, which results in distorted balance and possible injuries. To maintain good body balance while weight training, you must train both sides of your body equally.

Reduce body fat: Having too much non-value adding weight in your mid-section leads to several problems for baseball and softball players. This extra weight in your stomach disrupts your body's balance by causing you to unintentionally lean forward, putting stress on your lower back. Unfortunately, it is a physical impossibility to reduce fat exclusively from one area of the body, but a healthy diet, and proper weight training will reduce your body fat uniformly throughout your body.

Negative Effects of Excessive Body Fat

Aside from damaging your balance, excess body fat will negatively affect your speed and quickness, and will make you more injury prone. Carrying around unneeded fat wears down your muscles and fatigues your body. By carrying around this extra weight, your body will use up the energy you need to play, causing muscular and mental fatigue that can affect your game dramatically. One benefit of weight training is that it builds muscle mass, which increases the resting metabolism and reduces body fat.

Sometimes weight training alone is not enough to help you lose all of your unwanted fat, so it may be in your best interest to participate in a prolonged low-level aerobic activity such as walking, jogging, or riding the bike to complement your resistance training.

A Note to Coaches

Baseball and softball are anaerobic sports, requiring many short bursts of speed and no prolonged running. Having players do a lot of long-distance running during practice is not as beneficial as having them do sprints, which will build up their fast-twitch muscle fibers. A light jog to start out a practice is a good warm-up for players, but anything more than that may be a waste of practice time.

Off-Season Training

The off-season is the time in any sport to build up your muscles, become stronger, and more powerful. The off-season program consists of four different four-week routines cycled together to build both absolute strength and explosive power. The first and third routines are designed for you to put on size and strength while the second and fourth programs are designed for power and explosion.

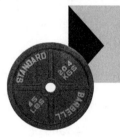

If you are interested in learning more about fast- and slow-twitch muscle fibers, refer to The Ultimate Guide to Weight Training for Sports.

Variation is one of the keys to a great workout program. The most important reason to vary your routines is so you can continue making progress and gains. Your body will eventually adapt to any routine it's on, so it is very important to change routines once your gains have stopped and your strength has peaked. Four weeks is the most effective time period to follow any one routine.

It cannot be stressed enough that during the off-season, you must supplement your weight-training activities with some sort of sport-specific activities to keep your body in proper shape. You must continue to practice your skills throughout the off-season to help keep your body loose and ready to play the next season.

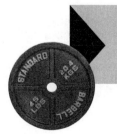

After following the first two 4-week off-season programs, be sure to take one week away from the gym to let your muscles rest and grow stronger before beginning your final two 4-week programs.

Strength Training

The stronger the vital areas of your body are, the better off you will be. Although some muscles are more important than others, every muscle in your body needs to be well trained. Five important aspects to strength training that the book provides:

Compound exercises: Each program contains many compound exercises, that is, an exercise (such as squats, bench presses, and lat pull downs) that trains two or more muscle groups. Most exercise and strength-training experts agree that compound exercises are the most efficient exercises for building strength and size.

Great form: For the best results, use great form while training. Take at least two seconds on the eccentric (negative) phase of the lift and at least one second on the concentric (positive) phase of the lift. This slow, rhythmic movement builds your muscles up bigger and stronger than any other type of lifting.

Pyramid Method: Several exercises in the strength-building routines are structured in a pyramid method of sets and reps, which is another strength-building tactic designed to maximize your efforts in the gym. When using the pyramid method, you decrease the reps and increase the load with every set. .

1

333

55555

Heavy weights, low reps: Building strength effectively requires lifting heavy weights between 1 and 8 repetitions for each set. Working to failure with fewer reps and heavier weights is the most effective way to put on strength and size quickly. To achieve the fastest and most effective results, train your muscles with the heaviest weights possible while still using good form. In most cases, people are able to lift heavier weights with barbells than dumbbells, which is why barbell exercises dominate strength programs. For optimal results, lift weights that are at least 85% of your one rep max.

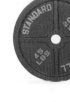

You can safely estimate your one rep max for any exercise using a one rep max calculator at www.sportsworkout.com

Extended rest time: By lifting such heavy weights, your muscles fatigue very quickly and need more rest time between sets than the other types of training. Generally two to five minutes between sets is ample time to rest. This rest time brings your heart rate back down closer to its resting rate so you are fully ready to complete another strenuous set with heavy weights.

Explosive-Power Training

The second and fourth routines of the cycle are designed to build speed and explosive power. Four important aspects to explosive power training are:

Medium weights, medium reps: Training for power is quite different than training for strength. For strength training, the idea is to lift heavy weights a low number of times. Contrastingly, decreasing the weight-load and lifting between eight and fifteen repetitions is the best way to successfully train for power and explosion.

Speed and intensity: With power training, the goal is to increase the speed while lifting. Before increasing the load, you want to increase the speed at which you are performing the concentric part, or positive phase of the lift. If the load begins to feel extremely light, then follow the steps listed in the section *When to Increase* located later in this book.

There are certain exercises, however, that should never be performed with speed and intensity due to the possibility of injury, or because fast movements are not as effective as slow ones. Exercises listed in our programs that should **never** be lifted with speed and intensity are:

1. Lower back exercises

2. Rotator cuff exercises

3. Mid-section exercises

Great Form: Similar to strength training, the lowering of the weight should be smooth and slow for at least two seconds. The difference comes on the concentric part of the lift. For power training you want to raise the weights as fast and explosively as possible. This works your fast-twitch muscle fibers with the goal of increasing the speed that you can contract and move your muscles. While following power-building routines, you are required to perform the concentric part of every rep in every set with intensity and speed. On a very important note, however, you must be sure to not sacrifice form for speed. Always make sure you perform the lift the proper way as instructed.

Power exercises: Certain exercises are most beneficial and most effectively performed with speed and intensity. Olympic lifts such as push presses and power cleans, as well as body weight exercises like dips, and pull-ups are such examples because they can be performed extremely fast with enormous amounts of intensity.

You will notice that a small number of low rep exercises for strength training are included to compliment the explosive power training. It is necessary that any explosive power weight-training program include at least some strength building aspects in order to maintain the strength you have acquired during the strength-training cycle. This ensures that upon completion of the first explosive power training routine, you will be able to start back up on the second strength-building program without losing any strength.

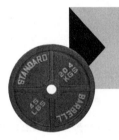

Remember to:
-Train your abs prior to each training session
-Stretch your muscles directly after each training session

Baseball and Softball Off-Season Program

Strength and Power Cycle
Weeks 1-4 Strength Training

Weeks 1-2

Days1 & 3

muscle group	exercise	sets	reps
shoulders	military	5	8,6,4,2,1
shoulders	standing flies	2	20,20
shoulders	bent over laterals	3	20,20,20
triceps	bench press	4	8,6,4,2
triceps	push downs	4	8,8,8,8
rotator cuff	prone	1	25
rotator cuff	side	1	25

Days2 & 4

muscle group	exercise	sets	reps
legs	leg Press	4	10,8,6,4
legs	leg Curl	4	10,8,6,4
back	wide grip pull downs	4	8,8,6,4
back	bent over rows	4	8,8,6,4
forearms	hammers	4	8,8,8,8
forearms	wrist curls	4	8,8,8,8
forearms	reverse wrist curls	4	8,8,8,8

Weeks 3-4

Days1 & 3

muscle group	exercise	sets	reps
shoulders	military	5	8,6,4,2,1
shoulders	lateral raises	3	20,20,20
shoulders	front raises	3	20,20,20
triceps	close grip bench	4	8,6,4,2
triceps	kick backs	4	8,8,8,8
rotator cuff	prone	1	25
rotator cuff	side	1	25

Days2 & 4

muscle group	exercise	sets	reps
legs	lunges	4	10,8,6,4
legs	calf raises	3	20,20,20
back	close grip pull downs	4	8,8,6,6
back	behind the neck pulls	4	8,8,6,6
forearms	reverse curls	4	8,8,8,8
forearms	wrist curls	4	8,8,8,8
forearms	reverse wrist curls	4	8,8,8,8

Weeks 5-8 Power Training

Weeks 5-6

Days1 & 3

muscle group	exercise	sets	reps
shoulders	push press	3	10,10,10
shoulders	cable lateral raises	3	12,12,12
shoulders	upright rows	3	12,12,12
triceps	dips	2	failure
triceps	bench dips	2	failure
rotator cuff	prone	1	25
rotator cuff	side	1	25

Days2 & 4

muscle group	exercise	sets	reps
legs	leg Press	4	10,8,6,4
legs	power clean	3	10,10,10
back	wide-grip pull-ups	2	failure
back	T bar rows	3	12,10,8
forearms	hammer curls	3	12,12,12
forearms	wrist curls	3	15,15,15

Weeks 7-8

Days1 & 3

muscle group	exercise	sets	reps
shoulders	push press	3	12,12,12
shoulders	standing flies	3	12,12,12
shoulders	lateral raises	3	15,15,15
triceps	dips	2	failure
triceps	close-grip bench press	4	15,12,8,4
rotator cuff	prone	1	failure
rotator cuff	side	1	failure

Days2 & 4

muscle group	exercise	sets	reps
legs	box step ups	3	10,10,10
legs	jump squat	3	10,10,10
back	close-grip pull ups	2	failure
back	one-arm dumbbell	3	12,12,12
forearms	wrist curls	3	15,15,15
forearms	reverse curls	3	15,15,15

Weeks 9-12 Strength Training

Weeks 9-10

Days1 & 3

muscle group	exercise	sets	reps
shoulders	military	5	8,6,4,2,1
shoulders	standing flies	2	20,20
shoulders	bent over laterals	3	20,20,20
triceps	bench press	4	8,6,4,2
triceps	push downs	4	8,8,8,8
rotator cuff	prone	1	25
rotator cuff	side	1	25

Days2 & 4

muscle group	exercise	sets	reps
legs	leg press	4	10,8,6,4
legs	leg curl	4	10,8,6,4
back	wide grip pull downs	4	8,8,6,4
back	bent over rows	4	8,8,6,4
forearms	hammers	4	8,8,8,8
forearms	wrist curls	4	8,8,8,8
forearms	reverse wrist curls	4	8,8,8,8

Weeks 11-12

Days1 & 3

muscle group	exercise	sets	reps
shoulders	military	5	8,6,4,2,1
shoulders	lateral raises	3	20,20,20
shoulders	front raises	3	20,20,20
triceps	close grip bench	4	8,6,4,2
triceps	kick backs	4	8,8,8,8
rotator cuff	prone	1	25
rotator cuff	side	1	25

Days2 & 4

muscle group	exercise	sets	reps
legs	lunges	4	10,8,6,4
legs	calf raises	3	20,20,20
back	close grip pull downs	4	8,8,6,6
back	behind the neck pulls	4	8,8,6,6
forearms	reverse curls	4	8,8,8,8
forearms	wrist curls	4	8,8,8,8
forearms	reverse wrist curls	4	8,8,8,8

Weeks 13-16 Power Training

Weeks 13-14

Days1 & 3

muscle group	exercise	sets	reps
shoulders	push press	3	10,10,10
shoulders	cable lateral raises	3	12,12,12
shoulders	upright rows	3	12,12,12
triceps	dips	2	failure
triceps	bench dips	2	failure
rotator cuff	prone	1	25
rotator cuff	side	1	25

Days2 & 4

muscle group	exercise	sets	reps
legs	leg press	4	10,8,6,4
legs	power clean	3	10,10,10
back	wide-grip pull-ups	2	failure
back	T bar rows	3	12,10,8
forearms	hammer curls	3	12,12,12
forearms	wrist curls	3	15,15,15

Weeks 15-16

Days1 & 3

muscle group	exercise	sets	reps
shoulders	push press	3	12,12,12
shoulders	standing flies	3	12,12,12
shoulders	lateral raises	3	15,15,15
triceps	dips	2	failure
triceps	close-grip bench press	4	15,12,8,4
rotator cuff	prone	1	failure
rotator cuff	side	1	failure

Days2 & 4

muscle group	exercise	sets	reps
legs	box step ups	3	10,10,10
legs	jump squat	3	10,10,10
back	close-grip pull ups	2	failure
back	one-arm dumbbell	3	12,12,12
forearms	wrist curls	3	15,15,15
forearms	reverse curls	3	15,15,15

Preseason Training

(Five weeks prior to the start of the season)

When the season begins, you need to be bursting with strength and explosive power. Our off-season program will have built you up an incredible base of both. Our preseason routine is designed to take you to the next level, to make you as strong and powerful as you can become leading right up to the season. Our preseason routine requires the eccentric part of the lift to remain slow and smooth while the concentric part of every rep to be done fast and with intensity and bursting explosion for power. You will notice that as the weeks progress, the number of reps required decreases and the weight increases. This is to ensure hardcore strength training to coincide with the power training. This style of lifting blends both strength and explosive power training together. The structure of the program is for strength, but your form will be for power.

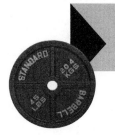

Remember to: -Train your abs prior to each training session
-Stretch your muscles directly after each training session

Preseason Training

Purpose: Endurance, Power, and Strength

Style: Holistic Training

Frequency: Two-day split, four days per week

Reps and Sets

Weeks 1 and 2:	sets of 10 reps
Weeks 3 and 4:	sets of 8 reps
Week 5:	sets of 6 reps

Day 1

muscle group	exercise	sets
shoulders	standing flies	3
shoulders	front raises	3
shoulders	lateral raises	3
rotator cuff	prone	3
forearms	reverse curls	1

Day 2

muscle group	exercise	sets
legs	leg press	3
legs	box steps	3
back	dumbbell rows	3
back	wide grip pull downs	3
rotator cuff	side	3
triceps	close grip bench	1

Day 3

muscle group	exercise	sets
shoulders	upright rows	3
shoulders	cable lateral raises	3
shoulders	barbell military press	3
rotator cuff	side	3
forearms	hammer curls	1

Day 4

muscle group	exercise	sets
legs	lunges	3
legs	jump squats	3
back	seated rows	3
back	close grip pull downs	3
rotator cuff	prone	3
triceps	dips	2

In-Season Training

Maintenance Training

While in season, the preferred method of training is for maintenance. The goal of in-season weight training is to maintain the gains you have acquired during the off-season, while being careful not to over train and become stale. When you become stale, your abilities and performance as an athlete decrease drastically. Lifting weights more than twice a week and practicing on a daily basis is more than enough to over train many people.

In order to maintain the endurance and explosion added in the off-season, in-season maintenance training calls for working out your major sport-specific muscle groups two days a week. This type of training is twice a week because it is the least number of days required to lift while still maintaining your gains. Training your muscles only once a week can cause them to lose the gains that they have acquired. The in-season routine includes maintenance exercises for endurance, strength, and explosive power elements so that nothing is lost during the season. If you wish, you can perform the in-season routine using a *circuit training* format. For more information on circuit training, see the *Training Techniques* section.

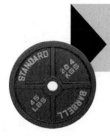

Remember to: -Train your abs prior to each training session
-Stretch your muscles directly after each training session

Odd Weeks

Day 1

muscle group	exercise	sets
shoulders	push press (jerks)	4
shoulders	standing flyes	3
chest	incline barbell bench press	4
back	close-grip pull downs	3
triceps	close-grip bench press	3

Day 2

muscle group	exercise	sets
legs	leg press	4
legs	leg curls	4
forearms	hammer curls	4
forearms	wrist curls	4

Even Weeks

Day 1

muscle group	exercise	sets
shoulders	barbell military press	4
shoulders	lateral raises	4
chest	barbell bench press	4
back	wide-grip pull downs	4
triceps	dips	2

Day 2

muscle group	exercise	sets
legs	dead lift	4
legs	lunges	4
forearms	reverse curls	4
forearms	wrist curls	4

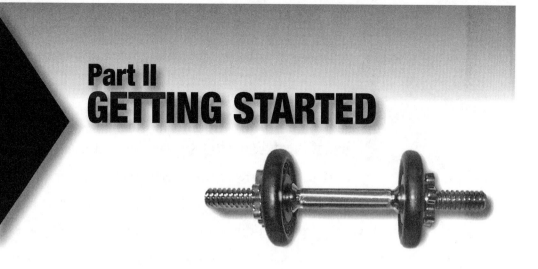

Part II
GETTING STARTED

Warming Up

Warming up is an essential part of a weight-training routine. *A warm-up activity can be any type of low-level activity as long as it loosens up your body, gets your blood flowing, and prepares your body for the workout.* Warming up is absolutely necessary if you plan to lift heavy weights. To walk into the gym and attempt to *max out* (lift the maximum amount of weight you can handle) without first warming up can cause injury because your body is not ready for the physical stress of a weight-training routine. In general, there are two major types of warming up, which are listed below.

A **full body warm-up** is anything that increases your blood flow and literally warms you up. Examples of full-body warm-up activities include low-intensity activities such as jogging or riding the bike for five to ten minutes prior to lifting weights. Other examples include about five to ten minutes of an abdominal routine, swimming a few laps, or even some full-body stretching.

An **exercise-specific warm-up** is properly executed by performing a light-weight *set* (group of repetitions) of an exercise before going into your prescribed routine for that same exercise with heavier weights. Ten repetitions are usually enough for a warm-up set. Basing your exercise-specific warm-up set on half of your *one-rep max* is the best technique. Your one-rep max is the maximum weight you can lift one time. Performing an exercise-specific warm-up increases your blood flow to the *active muscles*, that is, the muscles you are using.

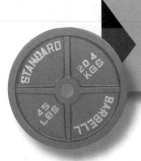

Warm-up sets should be performed with weights that are about half of your one-rep max. To determine your one rep max, log on to **www.sportsworkout.com** and use the one-rep max calculator.

Benefits of Warming Up One major benefit of warming up is that it helps reduce the likelihood of pulls, tears, and other injuries, which can be painful and hamper your future training. Another major benefit of warming up is that it loosens your muscles and allows you to lift heavier weights. Heavier weights, in turn, put more resistance on your muscles, which forces you work to harder and gives you a better workout.

Cooling Down

Cooling-down activities come directly after your weight-training session. While cooling down, the goal is, again, to loosen up your muscles. In this book, cool-down activities are synonymous with stretching exercises. Cooling-down activities are important because they can prevent soreness in the days following a weight-training session. They also increase your range of motion, helping you become more flexible, which can prevent injuries both in the weight room and in athletics. Because flexibility and range of motion are so important for all sports, stretching is a vital part of a complete workout program and should never be ignored.

There are numerous benefits to stretching and it is most effective during or after your workout. Stretching increases your range of motion and *stretching can be effective in injury reduction.* Proper stretching *may* also be effective in reducing soreness from weight training by helping to remove the anaerobic waste product—lactate—from your muscles.

Range of motion is essential for all sports and physical activities, and stretching is the way to increase it. It is a myth that weight training automatically makes you stiff and decreases your flexibility. Training *antagonistic*, or opposite, muscle groups in the same session actually stretches your muscles and helps increase your range of motion. An example of an antagonistic muscle group is the biceps and triceps. As the biceps contract, the triceps extend, which gives them a nice, full stretch.

Abs

Having a tight stomach, strong lower back, and incredible six-pack is important for several baseball and softball-related reasons. The exercises provided in this book will have you training properly and building picture-perfect abs. Lower back and oblique exercises are also incorporated with the abs routine so that your entire torso becomes stronger. Having strong abdominals is essential for high athletic performance. With tight abs and a strong lower back, you will be able to swing faster and more explosively. Your midsection connects your upper body to your lower body, and it allows you to apply the strength and power collectively in both areas.

By nature, the muscles in your midsection are different from the other muscles in your body and need to be trained differently in order to achieve maximum results. To train your abs properly, you need the following:

1. Slow movements: Abs are made up mostly of slow-twitch muscle fibers, which requires them to be trained with slow movements for optimal results. More information on slow- and fast-twitch fibers can be found in the section *Muscle Fibers*.

2. Quantity and consistency: Abdominals need to be trained for muscular endurance, not muscular strength, which requires many, many repetitions that can be performed daily.

3. Variety: Your midsection consists of different areas, each of which requires different exercises. To train each area, you need to perform a variety of exercises. Variety with any exercise is an essential part of muscle building and athletic training. Variety allows you to build and tone every part of the muscle you are training.

To keep things simple, this book refers to the areas of the abdomen as the:

- **Upper Abs**
- **Lower Abs**
- **Obliques**

Preferred Order of Training

Lower abs and oblique exercises are *compound exercises,* that is, they train more than one muscle group at a time. These exercises also train your upper abs. Upper abs exercises, on the other hand, strictly isolate your upper abs. In order to avoid fatigue in the upper abs, which are being worked in every type of abdominal exercise, and could prevent proper lower abs and obliques training, you should train the lower abs first, then the obliques, and lastly the upper abs.

The preferred order of training your abdominals is as follows:
- **Lower Abs**
- **Obliques**
- **Upper Abs**

Note: You can train your lower back before or after performing your abdominal exercises, depending on your personal preference.

Training your midsection for at least five minutes prior to lifting is a great way to warm up because you are both warming yourself up by increasing your blood flow, and you are also building and toning your entire midsection. This can be thought of this as killing two birds with one stone. Perform each exercise slowly and smoothly for one full minute without rest. Rest for 30 seconds between exercises.

Listed below are descriptions and pictures demonstrating exactly how to perform each of the recommended midsection exercises. Do not be overwhelmed by the vast number of recommended exercises. You only need to pick four or five of them for each warm-up routine. As your midsection becomes stronger, you should increase the number of exercises you perform so that you continue progressing in strength. Vary your routine constantly by choosing four or five different exercises to warm up with each day.

Abs Exercises

Definition: *Prime movers* are the muscles being directly trained in the exercise.

Standard Sit-ups

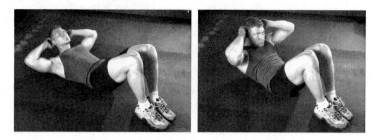

Prime Movers: Upper abs

Starting Position: Lie flat on your back with your knees bent and the soles of your feet flat on the floor. Elevate your tailbone about one inch above the floor. Place your hands on your ears.

Use your abs to lift the upper half of your body as high as you can, hold the position for a second or two, then slowly return to your starting position.

Tip: By keeping your tailbone elevated, you are working your lower abs, which is a target area for many people.

Standard Crunches

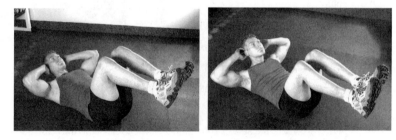

Prime Movers: Upper abs

Starting Position: Lie flat on your back with your feet and knees elevated so that your shins are parallel with the floor. Elevate your tailbone about one inch above the floor. Place your hands on your ears.

Use your abs to lift the upper half of your body. Once you've lifted your shoulders about thirty degrees off the floor, hold the position for a second or two, then slowly return to the starting position and repeat.

Oblique Crunches

Prime Movers: Obliques

Starting Position: Lie on your left side with your legs slightly bent, knees elevated about an inch or two above the floor, and your hands on your ears. Twist your torso to the right and do your best to keep your upper back and shoulders parallel with the floor.

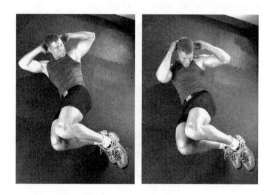

Use your obliques and upper abs to lift your upper body as high as you can and hold for a second or two. Return slowly to the starting position, and repeat. Then perform this exercise lying on your right side.

Tailbone Lifts

Prime Movers: Lower abs

Starting Position: Lie flat on your back
with your feet and knees elevated so that
your shins are parallel with the floor and
place your hands on your ears.

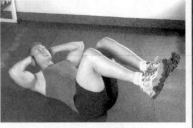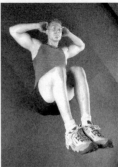

With your stomach flexed, use your lower abs to raise your tailbone an inch
or two off the floor. Hold that position for a second or two before lowering
your tailbone back to the floor. Be sure to keep your upper body in the same
position throughout the entire range of motion.

Elbow to Knee Sit-ups

Prime Movers: Entire torso

Starting Position: Lie flat on your back with
soles of your feet flat the floor. Place your
hands on your ears.

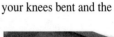 your knees bent and the

Use your abs to raise your upper
body forward while lifting your
left foot off the floor so that your

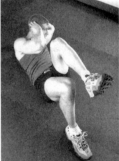

knee comes towards your head. Touch your knee to its opposite elbow.
Hold that position for a second or two with your abs flexed. Slowly lower
yourself back to the starting position and repeat the same movements with
your right knee and left elbow.

Bicycles

Prime Movers: Entire torso

Starting Position: Lie flat on your back with your knees bent, legs extended, feet elevated a few inches above the
floor, and your hands on your ears.

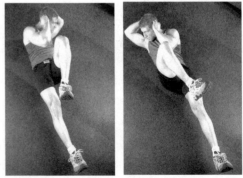

Use your abs to raise your upper body forward.
At the same time, begin to slowly pump your
legs one by one as if you were riding a bicycle.
As your knee comes towards to your head, touch
your raised knee to its opposite elbow. Hold that
position for a second or two with your abs flexed.
Go back to the starting point and repeat the same
movements with your other knee and elbow.

Side Bends

Prime Movers: Obliques

Starting Position: Standing upright, hold a dumbbell in your left hand and place your right hand on your head.

Lean your upper body a few inches to the left and use your obliques on the right side of your body to return to the starting position.

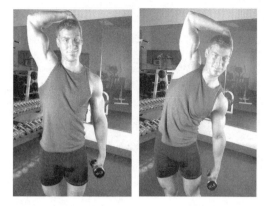

Good Mornings

Prime Movers: Lower back

Starting Position: Stand upright with your feet close together. Rest a barbell behind your neck on your traps. Keep your head tilted back and your back completely straight.

Slowly bend at the waist until you form a ninety-degree angle with your lower body. Slowly return to the starting position and repeat.

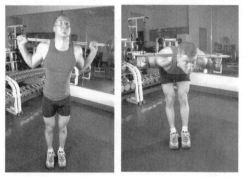

Hyperextensions

Prime Movers: Lower back

Starting Position: Lie face down on a hyperextension bench. Bend at the waist with your upper body hanging straight down and your hands placed behind your neck. Tilt your head back and keep your back straight.

Slowly raise your upper body until it is parallel with the floor and level with your lower body. Slowly return to the starting position and repeat.

Tip for hyperextensions and the preceding exercise, good mornings: Do not arch your back at any point because it can result in a painful injury

Reach Throughs

Prime Movers: Upper and lower abs

Starting Position: Lie flat on your back with your legs extended, slightly spread apart, and elevated a few

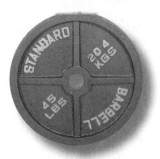

inches above the floor. Extend both your arms behind your head.

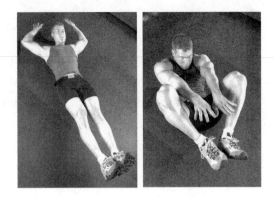

Use your abs to lift the upper half of your body up and bring your knees upward so that your shins are parallel with the floor. Simultaneously extend your arms directly in front of you, between your legs. Hold the position for a second or two, slowly return to the starting position, and repeat.

Leg Raises

Prime Movers: Lower abs

Starting Position: Lie on the floor with your legs extended and your shoulders and head tilted forward off the floor, putting stress on your upper abs. Place your hands underneath your tailbone to keep it slightly elevated above the floor. Keep your upper body stationary, hands underneath your tailbone, and legs locked throughout the entire range of motion.

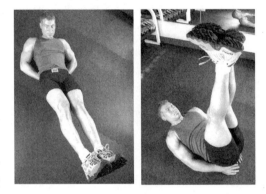

Raise your legs off the floor until they form a ninety-degree angle with the floor, allowing your tailbone and lower back to come off the floor in the process. Slowly lower your legs back to the starting position and repeat.

Tip: To get your legs that high may require a thrust from your abs, which in this case is okay.

Intercostal Pull Overs

Prime Movers: Intercostals

Starting Position: Lie on a bench with a barbell resting on your chest and your head slightly off the bench. Hold the bar with an overhand grip.

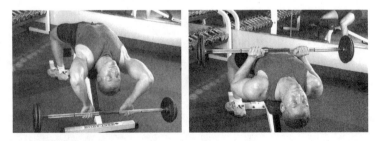

Slowly lift and lower the bar just over and behind your head until you feel a nice stretch in your chest. At this point raise the bar back over your head to the starting position.

Tip: If having your head partially off of the bench feels awkward and difficult, then perform this exercise with your head resting on the bench.

Stretching

Stretching is an absolutely crucial part to weight training for sports. It loosens you up, increases your range of motion, and may reduce the chance of injury and soreness in the days following a workout or athletic competition. Stretching is directly related to flexibility. This section goes into depth on how to properly stretch your muscles during or after a workout.

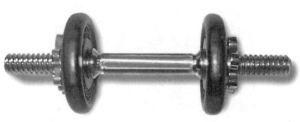

Everyone knows that stretching increases flexibility, but not everyone knows that lack of stretching decreases flexibility.

The recommended time for holding each stretch is ten seconds, resting thirty seconds between stretches. While holding a stretch, do not bounce; the stretch is less effective and can cause painful injuries. For every exercise, stretch as far as you can until you feel slight discomfort in the targeted areas. Go no farther once you reach that point. Hold that position for ten seconds as steadily as you can. Proper breathing and technique are extremely important. Do not hold your breath at any time during the stretch. The recommended stretching exercises and their descriptions and pictures are listed below.

Stretching Exercises

Hamstrings, Legs Crossed
Muscles stretched: Hamstrings.
> **Starting position**: Stand upright and cross your left foot over your right, keeping your legs straight. Bending at the waist, reach as far down as you can, and hold. Repeat with other leg.

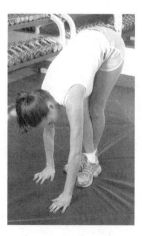

Hamstrings, Legs Spread

Muscles stretched: Hamstrings, groin.

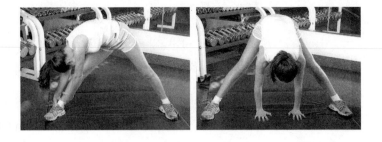

Starting Position: Stand upright and spread your legs slightly wider than shoulder width, keeping them straight.

Bending at the waist, reach as far down as you can to the outside leg and hold. Repeat to the other leg, then reach straight down. Rest between each stretch.

Hurdler Stretch

Muscles stretched: Hamstrings, quadriceps.

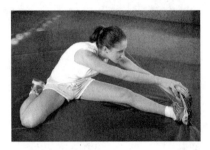

Starting Position: Sit on the floor with your right leg extended in front of you and your left leg bent at the knee and pointing behind you.

Bend at the waist and reach as far forward as you can to your right leg and hold.

Repeat with left leg extended.

Sit and Reach

Muscles stretched: Hamstrings, lower back.

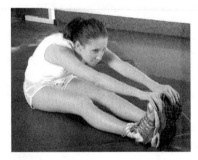

Starting Position: Sit on the floor with both legs extended in front of you.

Reach forward as far as you can towards your feet, and hold.

Standing Quad Stretch

Muscles stretched: Quadriceps.

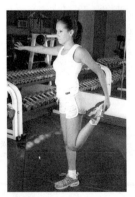

Starting Position: Stand upright on your left leg.

Grab your right ankle and pull it back as far as you can towards your buttocks and hold.

Repeat with other leg.

Neck Rolls

Muscles stretched: Neck.

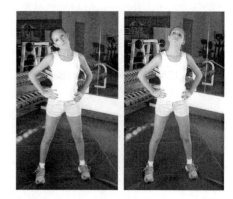

> **Starting Position:** Stand upright with your hands on your hips.
> Slowly roll your head clockwise in a circular motion using your full range of motion for ten rotations. Repeat going counterclockwise.

Across Body Arm Pulls

Muscles stretched: Shoulders, upper back.

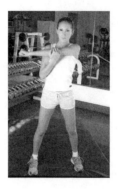

> **Starting Position:** Stand or sit upright with your back straight. Reach across your body with your left arm. Use your right hand to lightly pull and stretch the left arm as far and as close to your body as you can and hold. Repeat with other arm.

Overhead Arm Pulls

Muscles stretched: Triceps, shoulders, upper back.

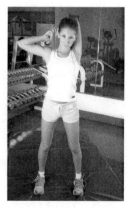

> **Starting Position:** Stand or sit upright with your back straight.
> Reach up and behind your neck with your left arm. Use your right hand to lightly pull and stretch your left arm as far as you can and hold.
> Repeat with other arm.

Butterflies

Muscles stretched: Groin, hips.

> **Starting Position**: Sit upright with your back straight and legs tucked in.

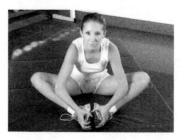

> Touch the soles of your shoes together and hold your toes with your hands. Pull your feet in as close as you can to your body.
> With your elbows, lightly push your knees towards the floor as far as you can and hold.

Seated Back Twists

Muscles stretched: Lower back, trunk, thighs, and hips.

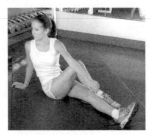

Starting Position: Sit upright with your back straight and left leg extended. Bend and cross your right leg over your left. Place your left forearm on the outside of your right leg, your right hand resting palm down on the floor next to you for balance. Twist your body to the right as far as you can and hold. Repeat to the other side.

Lying Knee Grabs

Muscles stretched: Glutes, hips.

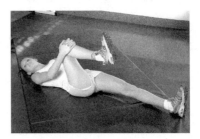

Starting Position: Lying flat on your back with your left knee bent and right leg extended, clasp your hands over the upper shin of your left knee.

Gently pull your left leg towards your chest until you feel the stretch and hold.

Repeat with other leg.

Standing Calves Stretch

Muscles stretched: Calves.

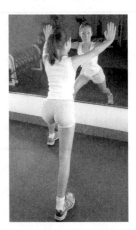

Starting Position: Stand leaning forward with your arms in front of you and your hands pushing against a wall. Place your left leg in front of the right.

Bend your left knee while keeping your right heel flat on the floor. Lean as far forward as you can while still keeping your back heel on the floor and hold.

Repeat with other leg.

Tip: This exercise also can be performed with both feet back.

Proper Form

Short- vs. Long-Term Results

In order to make the greatest gains in the least amount of time, you must perform each exercise properly. Lifting weights with bad form is very dangerous and can result in injury. Also, performing an exercise improperly is a waste of time in the gym. Though you may be able to lift heavier weights with improper form, your long-term results would suffer because you would not get as good a workout. You are better off working out for thirty minutes per day with excellent form and technique than lifting for three hours per day with improper form.

There are two movements to lifting a weight: the eccentric (negative) phase and the concentric (positive) phase.

The eccentric (negative) phase of the lift is the slow lowering of the weight. During this phase, your muscle is getting longer while still contracting. For example, in the bench press the eccentric phase occurs when you slowly lower the bar to your chest, lengthening your pectorals and triceps. Regardless of your purpose, the eccentric phase of the lift should always be slow and smooth, lasting at least two seconds. Always inhale while performing the eccentric phase of the lift.

> For the best results, the eccentric phase of every lift should last for at least two seconds.

The concentric (positive) phase of the lift is the exertion phase, or actual lifting of the weight. During this phase, the muscle shortens and the muscle cells contract. For example, in the bench press the concentric phase occurs when you lift the bar up from your chest so that your pectorals and triceps contract. The concentric phase of every lift should last at least one second unless you are training for power and explosion, where you lift the weight concentrically as fast as you can. Always exhale while performing the concentric phase of the lift.

Proper Breathing

DO NOT HOLD YOUR BREATH while lifting! Holding your breath can build up pressure in your body. Although extremely rare, if the pressure becomes extraordinarily intense, it can cut off blood circulation to your heart and brain. To avoid problems, just remember to breathe. Remember, you will get the most out of your lifting by inhaling on the eccentric part of the lift and exhaling while performing the concentric part of the lift.

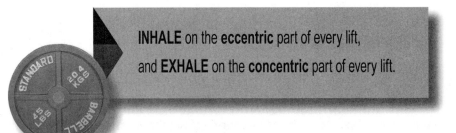

INHALE on the **eccentric** part of every lift,
and **EXHALE** on the **concentric** part of every lift.

Important note: If you have the determination to get to the gym for a set amount of time, then train with proper form and intensity so that you spend your time efficiently. Many people come home from the gym and feel a false sense of achievement simply because they had "made it to the gym." Once there, you need to work hard so you can *honestly* feel good about yourself for having taken one step closer to achieving your goals. Rather than going back to the gym over and over again to try and make up for lost time, do it right the first time.

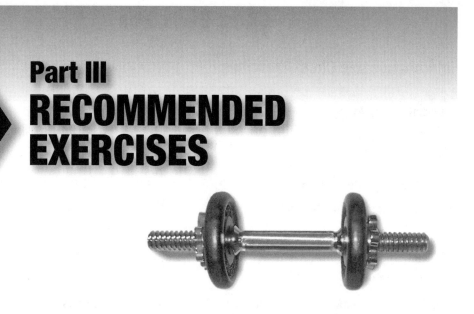

Part III
RECOMMENDED EXERCISES

This section provides you with every recommended weight-training exercise. You are given complete descriptions and pictures to ensure that you perform the exercises properly, safely, and effectively.

The numbers next to the exercises refer to their order of interchangeability, which is discussed in the following subsection. The muscles listed first after "prime movers" are the muscles that are being directly trained. Along with the descriptions are many helpful tips.

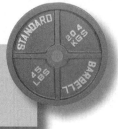

If you have any questions about anything in this book, be sure to e-mail **questions@sportsworkout.com** for help from certified personal trainers.

Substituting Similar Exercises

Our weight-training specialists did the hard work for you by strategically designing your program; all you have to do is follow it. Sometimes, however, there may be a required exercise or two that you either cannot perform physically or for which you do not have the equipment to perform. Many people struggle to do certain body weight exercises such as pull-ups or dips. Others may not have access to certain weight-training equipment such as cable or leg press machines. For these reasons, the exercises are listed for you are in order of interchangeability. If there is an exercise in your routine that you are not able to perform, substitute an exercise with a corresponding number from the same section. This substitution will ensure that you are training the same muscle groups in a similarly effective manner.

Chest Exercises

Interchangeable Chest Exercises

1 Barbell Bench Press

1 Dumbbell Bench Press

1 Pushups

2 Incline Barbell Bench Press

2 Incline Dumbbell Bench Press

3 Flyes

3 Incline Flyes

3 Cable Crossovers

Dips (can be interchanged with any chest, shoulder, or triceps exercise)

> **Safety tip!** When using a cable machine do not lower the weights so low or fast that they hit the weight stack. This stops the fluid motion of the lift and can cause injuries.

Barbell Bench Press

Prime movers: Chest, triceps, shoulders.

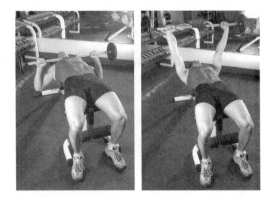

Starting Position: Lie on a flat bench with your feet flat on the floor. Keep your eyes directly below the bar and your hands shoulder width apart. Lift the bar off its supports until your arms are extended.

Lift:

a. Slowly lower the bar until it grazes you chest. The bar should come to a brief, complete stop.

b. Push the bar back to full extension with the bar directly in line with your chin.

Tip: Do not arch your back to try and lift more weight because it can cause serious back problems.

Tip: A closer grip trains your inner chest and triceps well; a wider grip works your outer chest.

Dumbbell Bench Press

Prime movers: Chest, triceps, shoulders.

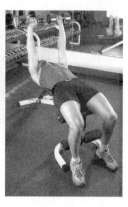

Starting Position: Lie on a flat bench with your feet flat on the floor. Hold the dumbbells with your arms extended.

Lift:

a. Slowly lower the dumbbells until you feel a comfortable stretch in your chest. The dumbbells should come to a brief, complete stop slightly below your chest.

b. Push the dumbbells back to full extension.

Tip: Dumbbells allow you to bring the weight lower than barbells, training your chest over the entire range of motion in ways a barbell cannot.

Pushups

Prime movers: Chest, shoulders, triceps.

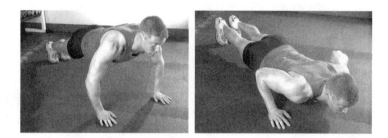

Starting Position: Lie face down on the floor with your back straight and palms on the floor, shoulder width apart, your legs locked, and your toes on the floor with your heels in the air.

Lift:

a. Push your body upward off of the floor until your arms are fully extended.

b. Slowly lower yourself until your chest is about an inch from the floor with your legs remaining locked. Come to a brief, complete stop before continuing.

Tip: To really train your triceps well, put your hands together and form a triangle with your index fingers and thumbs.

Incline Barbell Bench Press

Prime movers: Upper chest, triceps, shoulders.

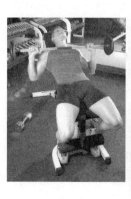
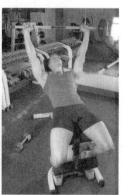

Starting Position: Lie on an inclined bench with your feet flat on the floor. Keep your eyes directly below the bar and your hands shoulder width apart.

Lift: Lift the bar off of its supports until your arms are extended.

a. Slowly lower the bar until it grazes your chest. The bar should come to a brief, complete stop.

b. Push the bar back to full extension with the bar directly in line with your chin.

Tip: You will not be able to lift as much as with a regular bench press. The steeper the degree of an incline, the less weight one typically is able to lift.

Incline Dumbbell Bench Press

Prime movers: Upper chest, triceps, shoulders.

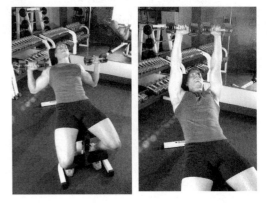

Starting Position: Lie on an inclined bench with your feet flat on the floor. Hold the dumbbells with your arms extended in the starting position.

Lift:

a. Slowly lower the dumbbells until you feel a comfortable stretch in your chest. The dumbbells should come to a brief, complete stop slightly below your chest.

b. Push the dumbbells back to full extension.

Flyes

Prime movers: Chest.

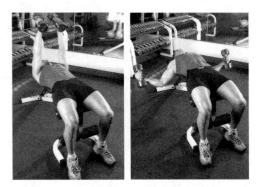

Starting Position: Lie on a bench with your feet flat on the floor. Hold the dumbbells with your arms extended and your palms facing each other so that the dumbbells are touching.

Lift:

a. Slowly lower the dumbbells away from each other with your arms slightly bent. Extend the dumbbells as wide as you can until you feel a comfortable stretch in your chest.

b. The dumbbells should come to a brief, complete stop slightly below your chest with your palms facing upward. Use your chest muscles to bring the dumbbells back to the starting position the same way they were brought down.

Tip: As you bring the dumbbells together, rotating your wrists and touching the tops and bottoms of the dumbbells together is a nice change of pace and trains your muscles from different angles.

Incline Flyes

Prime movers: Chest

Starting Position: Lie on an inclined bench with your feet flat on the floor. Hold the dumbbells with your arms extended and your palms facing each other so that the dumbbells are touching.

Lift:

a. Slowly lower the dumbbells away from each other with your arms slightly bent. Extend the dumbbells as wide as you can until you feel a comfortable stretch in your chest.

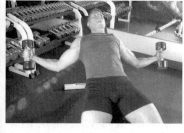
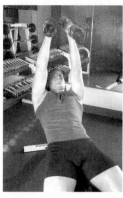

b. The dumbbells should come to a brief, complete stop slightly below your chest with your palms facing upward. Use your chest muscles to bring the dumbbells back to the starting position the same way they were brought down.

Cable Crossovers

Prime movers: Chest.

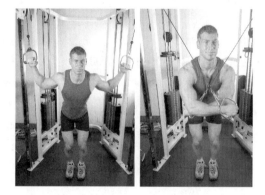

Starting Position: Stand bent slightly forward with your back straight and, with cables on both sides and slightly behind you, grab hold of the cables.

Lift:

a. With your arms slightly bent, use your chest to slowly bring the cables towards each other where they will pass each other in front of you. Cross the cables as far as you can.

b. The cables should come to a brief, complete stop. Then, slowly allow the cables to go back to the starting position the same way they were brought across.

Tip: Alternate which arm is on top and bottom for every rep to ensure both sides are getting equal training.

Dips

Prime movers: Chest, shoulders, triceps.

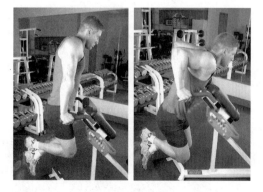

Starting Position: With arms extended, grip the parallel bars with both hands so that your body is elevated off the floor.

Lift:

a. With your elbows tucked in as closely as possible and your back straight, slowly lower yourself until your chin is parallel with the bars.

b. Use your chest muscles, shoulders, and triceps to push back up to full extension with your arms locked.

Tip: The farther you lean your body forward, the more your chest gets trained. As you straighten your body, your triceps begin to do the bulk of the work.

Back (Lats) Exercises

Interchangeable Back (Lats) Exercises

1 Lat Pull Downs

1 Behind-the-Neck Pull Downs

1 Seated Cable Rows

1 Pull-ups

2 Bent-Over Barbell Rows

2 Bent-Over Dumbbell Rows

2 T-bar Rows

2 One-Arm Dumbbell Rows

Lat Pull Downs

Prime movers: Lats, biceps, shoulders.

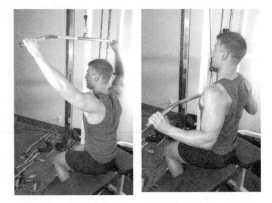

Starting Position: Sit at a lat pull down machine. Keep your back straight and lean backward a few inches with your feet resting on the floor. Grab the bar with both hands, using an overhand grip.

Lift:

a. Keeping your body stationary and bending at the elbows, pull the bar down in front of your neck, squeezing your shoulder blades together until the bar grazes your chest.

b. Let the bar come to a brief, complete stop before slowly and controllably guiding it back up to its original starting position, the same way you pulled it down.

Tip: This exercise can also be performed with an underhand grip.

> **Tip for all pull-downs and pull-ups:** The wider the grip, the more you train the upper part of your back. The closer the grip, the more you train the lower part of your back.

Behind-the-Neck Pull Downs:

Prime movers: Lats, shoulders, biceps.

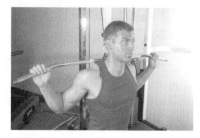

Starting Position: Sit upright at a lat pull down machine. Keep your back straight with your feet resting on the floor. Grab the bar with both hands, using an overhand grip.

Lift:

a. Keeping your body stationary and bending at the elbows, pull the bar down behind your neck, squeeze your shoulder blades together, and bring the bar as low as you can.

b. Let the bar come to a brief, complete stop before slowly and controllably guiding it back up to its original starting position, the same way you pulled it down.

Tip: More flexible people will be able to pull the bar down lower. Do not pull the bar down so low that it starts to feel uncomfortable. If you feel any unusual pain, DO NOT perform this exercise.

Seated Cable Rows

Prime movers: Lats, biceps, shoulders.

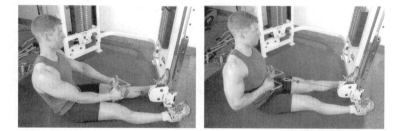

Starting Position:

Sit at a row machine with your back straight, feet resting on the foot rests and legs slightly bent. Lean forward and grab the handles.

Lift:

a. Keeping your back straight, lean backward and pull the handles towards your stomach as far back as you can, squeezing your shoulder blades together.

b. Let the handles come to a brief, complete stop before slowly and controllably guiding them back up to their original starting position, the same way you pulled them up.

Pull-ups

Prime movers: Lats, biceps, shoulders.

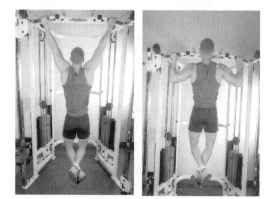

Starting Position: Grab hold of a pull-up bar using an overhand grip with your arms completely extended and feet crossed and off the floor.

Lift:

a. Keeping your body stationary, feet crossed, and bending at the elbows, pull your body up in front of the bar as high as you can, squeezing your shoulder blades together.

b. Let your body come to a brief, complete stop before slowly and controllably lowering it back down to its original starting position, the same way you pulled it up.

Tip: This exercise can also be performed behind the neck or with an underhand grip.

Tip: To train for optimal results, be sure to lower yourself all the way until your arms are nearly extended.

Bent-Over Barbell Rows

Prime movers: Lats, biceps, shoulders.

Starting Position: Standing with your knees slightly bent, feet a couple of inches apart, and bending at the waist to form an approximate ninety-degree angle, hold a bar with your arms hanging in front of you. Keep your back straight and your head tilted back.

Lift:

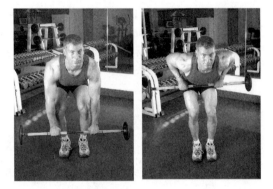

a. Keeping your body stationary and bending at the elbows, pull the bar up towards your stomach squeezing your shoulder blades together.

b. Let the bar come to a brief, complete stop before slowly and controllably guiding it back up to its original starting position, the same way you pulled it up.

Tip for all bent-over back exercises: Do not pull the weights towards your chest; this does not isolate your lats as well as raising the bar to your stomach.

Bent-Over Dumbbell Rows

Prime movers: Lats, biceps, shoulders.

Starting Position: Standing with your knees slightly bent, feet a couple of inches apart, and bending at the waist to form an approximate ninety-degree angle, hang your arms to the sides and hold two dumbbells with your palms facing each other. Keep your back straight and your head tilted back.

Lift:

a. Keeping your body stationary and bending at the elbows, pull the dumbbells up the sides of your body as high as you can, squeezing your shoulder blades together.

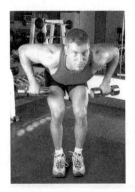

b. Let the dumbbells come to a brief, complete stop before slowly and controllably guiding them back up to their original starting position, the same way you pulled them up.

T-bar Rows

Prime movers: Lats, biceps, shoulders.

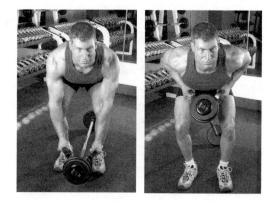

Starting Position: Standing with your knees slightly bent, feet a couple of inches apart, and bending at the waist to form a forty-five-degree angle with your floor, use an overhand grip to hold the handles of a T-bar machine, keeping the weights off of the floor. Keep your back straight and your head tilted back.

Lift:

a. Keeping your body stationary and bending at the elbows, pull the bar up towards your chest squeezing your shoulder blades together.

b. Let the bar come to a brief, complete stop before slowly and controllably guiding it back up to its original starting position, the same way you pulled it up.

Tip: If no T-bar machines are available, you can make your own using a barbell and a cable bar, as shown in the picture.

One-Arm Dumbbell Rows

Prime movers: Lats, biceps, shoulders.

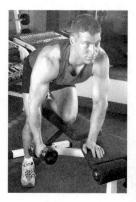

Starting Position: Standing with your left hand and left knee resting on a bench, bend at the waist to form an approximate ninety-degree angle. Hang your right arm to the side and hold the dumbbell with your palm facing towards your body. Keep your back straight and your head tilted back.

Lift:

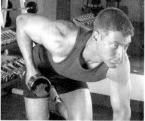

a. Keeping your body stationary and bending at the elbow, pull the dumbbell up the side of your body as high as you can.

b. Let the dumbbell come to a brief, complete stop before slowly and controllably guiding it back up to its original starting position, the same way you pulled it up.

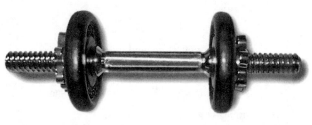

Shoulders Exercises

Interchangeable Shoulder Exercises

1 Barbell Military (Shoulder) Press
1 Dumbbell Military (Shoulder) Press
1 Push Press (Jerks)
2 Front Raises
2 Lateral Raises
2 Bent-Over Lateral Raises
2 Cable Lateral Raises
3 Standing Flyes
3 Upright Rows
4 Barbell Shrugs
4 Dumbbell Shrugs
5 Rotator Cuff Prone Position
5 Rotator Cuff On Side

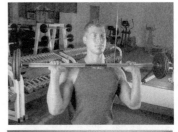

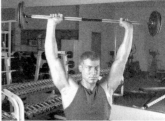

Barbell Military (Shoulder) Press

Prime movers: Shoulders, triceps.

Starting Position: Stand or sit upright and hold a bar at your shoulders, using an overhand grip. Grip the bar with your hands slightly wider than shoulder width.

Lift:

a. Keeping your body still, push the bar straight up until your arms are extended.

b. Slowly lower the bar down to the original starting position.

Dumbbell Military (Shoulder) Press

Prime movers: Shoulders, triceps.

Starting Position: Stand or sit upright and hold dumbbells at your shoulders. Hold them with your hands slightly wider than shoulder width.

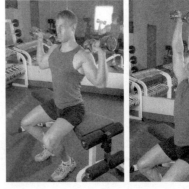

Lift:

a. Keeping your body still, push the dumbbells straight up until your arms are extended.

b. Slowly lower the dumbbells down to their original starting position.

Push Press (Jerks)

Prime movers: Shoulders, triceps, legs.

Starting Position: Stand with your back straight and knees slightly bent. Hold the bar at your shoulders using an overhand grip. Grip the bar with your hands slightly wider than shoulder width.

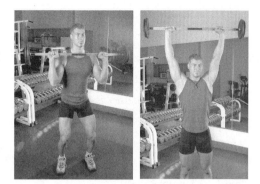

a. Explode upwards with your legs to give the bar some upward momentum. With this momentum, push the bar straight up until your arms are extended.

b. Slowly lower the bar down and return to the starting position.

Front Raises

Prime movers: Shoulders, traps.

Starting Position: Stand or sit upright and hold two dumbbells in front of you with your palms facing towards your body.

Lift:

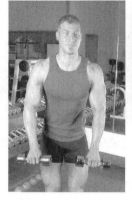

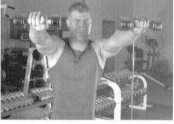

a. With your arms remaining straight, raise the dumbbells out in front of you in one smooth, fluid motion until your hands are slightly above your shoulders.

b. Let the dumbbells come to a brief, complete stop before slowly lowering them back down to their original starting position, the same way you raised them up.

Lateral Raises

Prime movers: Shoulders, traps.

Starting Position: Stand or sit upright and hold two dumbbells at your sides with your palms facing your body.

Lift:

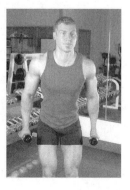

Tip for all shoulder raises: Once you raise your arms beyond a ninety-degree angle with your body, you begin to focus more on your traps.

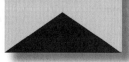

a. With your arms remaining straight, raise the dumbbells out to your sides in one smooth, fluid motion until your hands are slightly above your shoulders and slightly in front of you. As they reach this position, rotate your thumbs downward as if you are pouring a glass of water.

b. Let the dumbbells come to a brief, complete stop before slowly lowering them back down to their original starting position, the same way you raised them up.

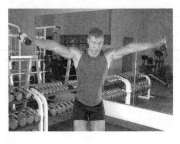

Tip: This exercise can also be performed with your palms pointing upward towards the ceiling.
Tip for all shoulder raises: You can raise the dumbbells with both arms at the same time or alternate arms.

Bent-Over Lateral Raises

Prime movers: Shoulders, traps.

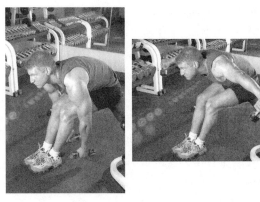

Starting Position: Stand or sit bent at the waist, keeping your back completely straight and forming a ninety-degree angle with your legs. Let your arms hang straight down in front of you with your palms facing each other.

Lift:

a. With your arms remaining straight, raise your arms out to your sides until they are parallel with your shoulders and slightly in front of you. As they reach shoulder level, rotate your thumbs downward in one smooth, fluid motion as if you are pouring a glass of water.

b. Let the dumbbells come to a brief, complete stop before slowly lowering them back down to their original starting position the same way you raised them up.

Cable Lateral Raises

Prime movers: Shoulders, traps.

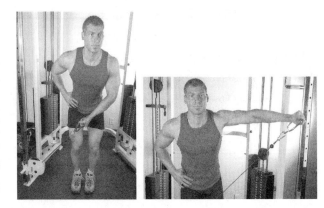

Starting Position: Stand with your right arm next to a cable machine with your back straight. Grab hold of the cable with your left arm, so that your arm is hanging, slightly bent, across the front of your body. Rest the hand you are not using on your hip.

Lift:

a. Keeping your body still and your arm slightly bent, raise the cable across your body and out to the side in one motion until your hand is elevated slightly above your shoulder. As it reaches this level, rotate your thumbs downward in one smooth, fluid motion as if you are pouring a glass of water.

b. Let the cable come to a brief, complete stop before slowly lowering it back down to its original starting position the same way you raised it up.

Standing Flyes

Prime movers: Shoulders, traps.

Starting Position: Stand upright or with your knees slightly bent and bend at the waist with your back straight to form a forty-five-degree angle with your lower body. With your palms facing each other, hold two dumbbells a few inches in front of your chest with your elbows bent at ninety-degree angles.

Lift:

a. Keeping your body still and your arms bent at 90-degree angles, pull the weights upward and backward as far back as you can, squeezing your shoulder blades together.

b. Come to a brief, complete stop before slowly returning the weights back to their starting position the same way you raised them up.

> **Tip for standing flyes and upright rows:** Avoid using your back and body momentum to complete these lifts because doing so is not an effective way of training and could cause injury.

Upright Rows

Prime movers: Shoulders, traps, biceps.

Starting Position: Stand upright with your arms hanging in front of you. Hold a barbell with an overhand grip. Your hands should be roughly eight inches apart.

Lift:

a. Keeping your body still and back straight, raise the bar upwards to your chin, keeping the bar as close to your body as you can without touching it.

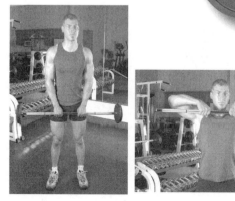

b. Let the bar come to a brief, complete stop before slowly lowering it back down to its original starting position the same way you raised it up.

Barbell Shrugs

Prime movers: Traps

Starting Position: Stand upright 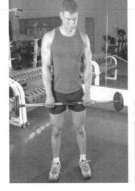 with your arms hanging in front of you. Hold a barbell with an overhand grip, hands roughly shoulder-width apart.

Lift:

a. Keeping your body still, back straight, and arms hanging in front of you, raise only your shoulders straight up.

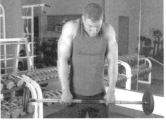

b. Hold the position for at least three seconds before slowly lowering your shoulders back down to the original starting position.

Dumbbell Shrugs

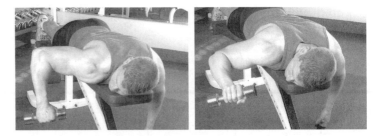

Tip for barbell and dumbbell shrugs: Keeping your head down increases your range of motion for these exercises, giving your traps a better workout.

Prime movers: Traps

Starting Position: Stand upright with arms hanging at your sides. Hold dumbbells with your palms facing each other.

Lift:

a. Keeping your body still, back straight, and arms hanging at your sides, raise only your shoulders straight up.

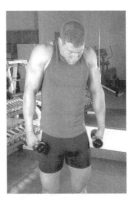

b. Hold the position for at least three seconds before slowly lowering your shoulders back down to the original starting position.

Rotator Cuff Prone Position

Area trained: Rotator cuff.

Starting Position:

Lie face down on a bench with one arm extended to the side so that your upper arm is parallel to the floor. Bend your arm at a ninety-degree angle so that your hand is hanging with your palm facing behind you. Hold a light weight in that hand.

Lift:

a. Keeping everything else stationary, rotate your forearm upward until it becomes parallel with the ground.

b. Slowly lower the weight back to its original starting position, the same way you brought it up.

> **Tip:** All rotator cuff exercises should always be performed very slowly and smoothly, and the weights for these exercises should **NEVER** exceed three lbs. or injuries will occur.

Rotator Cuff on Side

Area trained: Rotator cuff.

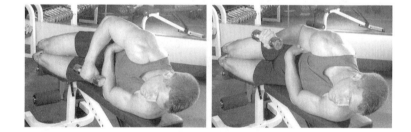

Starting Position:

Lie on your side on a bench with your upper arm resting on your chest, parallel to the floor, and bent at the elbow at a ninety-degree angle so that your hand is hanging. Hold a light weight in that hand.

Lift:

a. Keeping everything else stationary, rotate your arm upward until it becomes parallel with the ground.

b. Slowly lower the weight back to its original starting position, the same way you brought it up.

Triceps Exercises

Interchangeable Triceps Exercises

1 Triceps Push Downs

1 Triceps Pull Downs

1 Skull Crushers

1 Triceps Kickbacks

1 Bench Dips

2 Barbell Triceps Curls

2 Dumbbell Triceps Curls

2 One-Arm Triceps Extensions

Triceps Push Downs

Prime movers: Triceps.

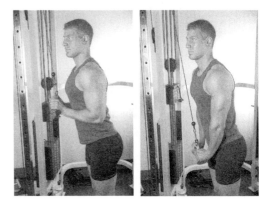

Starting Position: Stand or kneel with your back straight in front of a cable machine. Grab the bar with an overhand grip. Keep your elbows tucked in at your sides and hold the bar up by your chin.

Lift:

a. Keeping your body still and elbows tucked at your sides, push the bar straight down until your arms are fully extended.

b. Come to a brief, complete stop before slowly allowing the bar to rise back up to the starting position, with your elbows remaining tucked at your sides at all time.

Tip: For variation, you can use many types of bars, including one-arm handles.

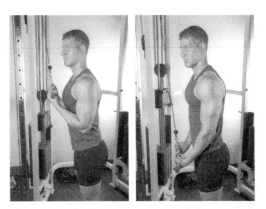

Triceps Pull Downs

This exercise is identical to triceps push downs with an underhand grip.

Skull Crushers

Prime movers: Triceps.

Starting Position: Lie on a bench with your head partially hanging off the end. Hold a barbell with a close overhand grip straight out in front of you, above your forehead, with your arms extended.

Lift:

a. Keeping your body still and elbows motionless, slowly lower

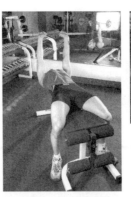

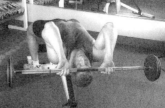

your forearms and the barbell down behind your head as far as you can.

b. Come to a brief, complete stop before returning the barbell to the starting position the same way you brought it down. Keep your elbows in and do not use your shoulders.

Tip: If having your head partially off of the bench feels awkward and difficult, then perform this exercise with your head resting on the bench.

> If balance becomes an issue while performing any cable machine triceps exercise, stand stagger stepped, with one leg behind the other.

Triceps Kickbacks

Prime movers: Triceps.

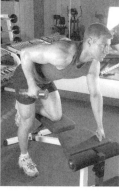
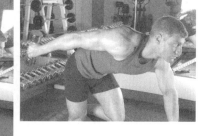

Starting Position: Stand bending at the waist so your upper body is parallel with the floor with your knees slightly bent. Stand stagger stepped or place one knee on a bench and place your opposite hand on a bench for balance. With your elbow tucked in at your side and your upper arm also parallel to the floor, let your lower arm hang down perpendicular to the floor.

Lift:

a. Keeping your body still and elbow motionless, raise your lower arm backward until your arm is fully extended.

b. Come to a brief, complete stop before slowly lowering the dumbbell to the starting position, the same way you brought it up. Keep your elbow in and do not use your shoulder.

Bench Dips:

Prime movers: Triceps, shoulders.

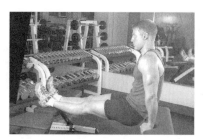

Starting Position: Place your heels on one bench in front of you and your palms on another bench behind you shoulder-width, leaving your rear hanging in the air.

Your heels should be together and your hands should be shoulder-width apart. Your arms should be extended so that your body is elevated.

Lift:

a. Slowly lower yourself by bending at the elbows as low as you can by keeping the elbows tucked in as much as possible and keeping your back straight.

b. Push yourself back up to full extension with your arms locked.

Tip: If your body weight alone is not providing enough resistance for a good workout, try placing some weights on your lap.

Barbell Triceps Curls

Prime movers: Triceps.

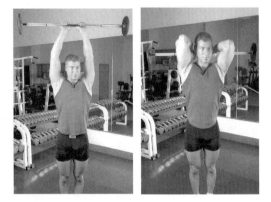

Starting Position: Stand or sit upright and hold a barbell above your head with your arms locked out and your elbows close to your head.

Lift:

a. Keeping your body still and elbows fixed close to your head, slowly lower your forearms and the bar down behind your head as far as you can.

b. Come to a brief, complete stop before returning the bar to the starting position, the same way you brought it down. Keep your elbows in and do not use your shoulders.

Tip: Keeping your elbows in close to your head is sometimes difficult to do, but it ensures the best triceps workout.

Dumbbell Triceps Curls:

Prime movers: Triceps.

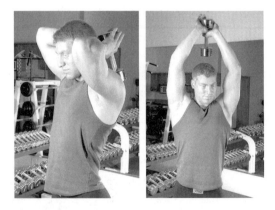

Starting Position: Stand or sit upright and hold a dumbbell above your head with both hands, your arms locked out, and your elbows close to your head.

Lift:

a. Keeping your body still and elbows fixed close to your head, slowly lower your forearms and the dumbbell down as far as you can.

b. Come to a brief, complete stop before returning the dumbbell to the starting position, the same way you brought it down. Keep your elbows in and do not use your shoulders.

One-Arm Triceps Extensions:

Prime movers: Triceps.

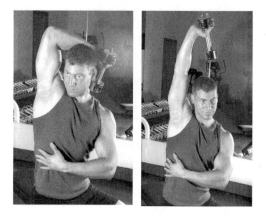

> **Starting Position:** Stand or sit upright and hold a dumbbell above your head with one hand. Keep your arm locked out and your elbow close to your head.
>
> **Lift:**
>
> **a.** Keeping your body still and elbow fixed close to your head, slowly lower your forearm and the dumbbell down behind your head as far as you can.
>
> **b.** Come to a brief, complete stop before returning the dumbbell to the starting position, the same way you brought it down. Keep your elbow in and do not use your shoulder.

Biceps/Forearms Exercises

Interchangeable Biceps/ Forearms Exercises

1 Barbell Curls

1 Dumbbell Curls

1 Preacher Curls

1 Incline Dumbbell Curls

1 Concentration Curls

2 Reverse Barbell Curls

2 Reverse Dumbbell Curls

2 Hammer Curls

3 Behind Back Wrist Curls

3 Reverse Wrist Curls

Barbell Curls

Prime movers: Biceps.

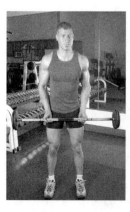
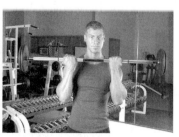

> **Starting Position:** Stand upright with your feet roughly shoulder-width apart. Hold a barbell with your palms facing away from your body and elbows tucked into your sides.

Lift:

a. Keeping your elbows tucked at your sides at all times, use your biceps to curl the bar upward as high as you can until it is just below your chin.

b. With your elbows still tucked at your sides, slowly lower the bar back to its original starting position.

Tip: Performing cheat curls (allowing your body to rock backward slightly to gain momentum) with this exercise from time to time can be beneficial to gaining mass in the biceps. You MUST wear a weight-lifting belt if you perform cheat curls. .

Dumbbell Curls

Prime movers: Biceps.

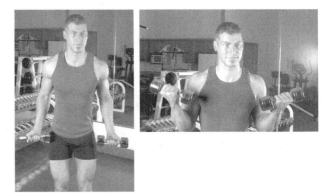

Starting Position: Stand or sit upright and with your feet roughly shoulder-width apart, hold dumbbells with your palms facing away from your body and elbows tucked into your sides.

Lift:

a. Keeping your elbows tucked at your sides at all times, use your biceps to curl the dumbbells upward as high as you can. You can curl with both arms at the same time or alternate arms.

b. With your elbows still tucked at your sides, slowly lower the bar back to its original starting position.

Tip for all dumbbell biceps exercises: Rotating your wrists inward towards your body will add extra emphasis and will give your biceps an even greater peak.

Preacher Curls

Prime movers: Biceps.

Starting Position: Sit at a preacher bench with your elbows resting on the bench shoulder-width apart. Grip the bar with your palms facing upward.

Lift:

a. With your elbows remaining stationary, use your biceps to curl the bar upward as high as you can towards your chin, where you should flex your biceps for extra emphasis.

b. Slowly lower the bar back to its original starting point with your arms full extended.

Tip: A closer grip trains your outer biceps and a wider grip trains your inner biceps.

Incline Dumbbell Curls

Prime movers: Biceps.

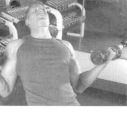

Starting Position: Sit on an inclined bench with your elbows tucked at your sides and your arms fully extended. Grip the dumbbells with your palms facing upward.

Lift:

a. Keeping your elbows tucked at your sides at all times, use your biceps to curl the dumbbells upward as high as you can. You can curl with both arms at the same time or alternate arms.

b. With your elbows still tucked at your sides, slowly lower the bar back to its original starting position.

Concentration Curls

Prime movers: Biceps.

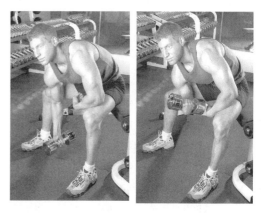

Starting Position: Sit on a bench slightly bent forward with your left arm gripping a dumbbell hanging between your legs. Your left palm should face your right leg and your right arm should rest on your knee.

Lift:

a. Keeping your elbow and upper arm stationary, curl the weight upward towards your shoulder.

b. With your elbow and upper arm still stationary, slowly lower the bar back to its original starting position.

Reverse Barbell Curls

Prime movers: Forearms, biceps.

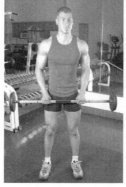
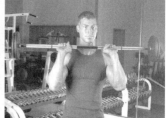

Starting Position: Stand upright with your feet roughly shoulder-width apart. Hold a barbell with your palms towards your body, your wrists locked, and elbows tucked into your sides.

Lift:

a. Keeping your elbows tucked at

your sides and wrists locked at all times, use your forearms and biceps to curl the bar upward as high as you can or until it is just below your chin.

b. With your elbows still tucked at your sides, slowly lower the bar back to its original starting position.

Tip: Keeping your wrists locked adds extra emphasis to your forearms and ensures a great workout.

Reverse Dumbbell Curls

Prime movers: Forearms, biceps.

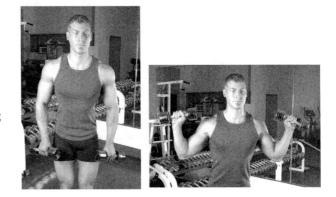

Starting Position: Stand or sit upright with your feet roughly shoulder-width apart. Hold two dumbbells with your palms facing towards your body, your wrists locked, and elbows tucked into your sides.

Lift:

a. Keeping your elbows tucked at your sides and wrists locked at all times, use your forearms and biceps to curl the dumbbells upward as high as you can. You can curl with both arms at the same time or alternate arms.

b. With your elbows still tucked at your sides and wrists locked, slowly lower the bar back to its original starting position.

Hammer Curls

Prime movers: Forearms, biceps.

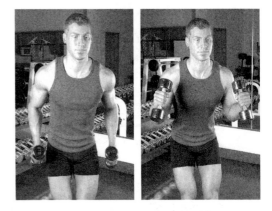

Starting Position: Stand or sit upright with your feet roughly shoulder-width apart. Hold two dumbbells with your palms facing each other, your wrists locked, and elbows tucked into your sides.

Lift:

a. Keeping your elbows tucked at your sides, wrists locked, and palms facing each other at all times, use your forearms and biceps to curl the dumbbells upward as high as you can. You can curl with both arms at the same time or alternate arms.

b. With your elbows still tucked at your sides, wrists locked, and palms facing each other, slowly lower the dumbbells back to their original starting position.

Behind Back Wrist Curls

Prime movers: Forearms.

Starting Position: Stand upright with your feet roughly shoulder-width apart. Hold a barbell behind your back as if you are handcuffed with your palms facing away from your body and elbows tucked into your sides.

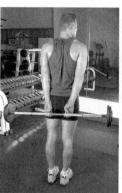
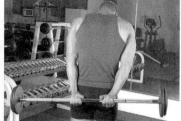

Lift:

a. Keeping your elbows tucked at your sides at all times, use your wrists to curl the bar upward towards your forearms.

b. With your elbows still tucked at your sides, slowly lower the bar with your wrists back to its original starting position.

Reverse Wrist Curls

Prime movers: Forearms.

Starting Position: Sit at the end of a bench. Hold a barbell with an overhand grip with your palms facing the floor and your forearms resting on your thighs.

Lift:

a. Keeping everything stationary, use your wrists to curl the bar backwards as far as you can.

b. Slowly lower the bar with your wrists, back to its original starting position.

Legs Exercises

Interchangeable Leg Exercises

1 Squats

1 Leg Press

1 Dead Lift

1 Leg Extensions

1 Leg Curls

2 Standing Calf Raises

2 Seated Calf Raises

2 Reverse Calf Raises

3 Jump Squats

3 Power Cleans

4 Box Steps

4 Lunges

Squats

Prime movers: Upper and lower legs.

Starting Position: Stand upright with your feet shoulder-width apart and a barbell resting behind your neck on your traps with your hands slightly wider than shoulder-width apart, using an overhand grip. Keep your back straight and your head tilted up.

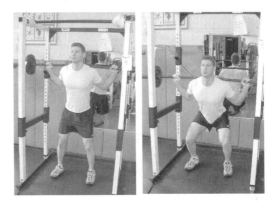

Lift:

a. With your back remaining straight and your head tilted up, slowly lower the weight by bending your knees until the upper part of your legs is parallel with the floor.

b. Explode upward back to the starting position. The entire lift should be in one smooth, fluid motion.

> **Tip for squats and dead lifts:** Standing up on your toes as high as you can and holding it for a second or so upon returning to the starting position is a great built-in calves workout.

Leg Press

Prime movers: Upper and lower legs.

Starting Position: Sit in a leg press machine with your back straight. Place your hands on the handlebars and your feet on the support bar.

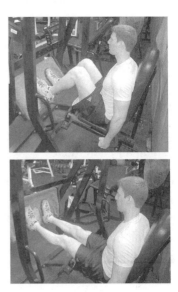

Lift:

a. With everything remaining still, slowly lower the weight by bending your knees as far as you can.

b. Explode upward back to the starting position. The entire lift should be in one smooth, fluid motion.

Tip: By not lowering the weights down very far, you are able to lift more weights, but will not be training your legs through the entire range of motion.

Dead Lift:

Prime movers: Upper and lower legs.

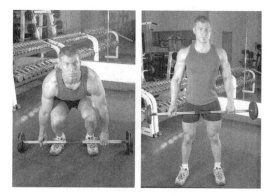

Starting Position: Stand with your back straight, head tilted back, and leaning slightly forward at the waist. Bend your knees so you can grab a barbell with your arms fully extended.

a. Keeping your arms locked, push with your legs to an upright position. Your lower back will also be used, but try to concentrate on using only your legs to lift the bar off the floor.

b. Slowly lower the bar so that it comes a few inches from the floor, with your arms and back remaining straight and head tilted up.

Tip: You may find this exercise easier to perform by gripping the bar with one hand using an overhand grip and the other hand using an underhand grip as shown in the pictures.

Leg Extensions

Prime movers: Quadraceps.

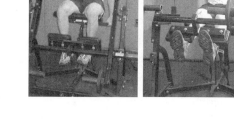

Starting Position: Sit with your back straight and hands gripping the handlebars in a leg-extension machine. Place your feet underneath the bar.

Lift:

a. With everything remaining still, raise the bar with your feet by extending your legs as far as you can.

b. Slowly lower your legs back down towards the starting position the same way you brought them up.

Tip: If all of the weights on your leg extension/curl machine are still not enough for you, you can perform this exercise one leg at a time.

Leg Curls

Prime movers: Hamstrings.

Starting Position: With your back straight and hands gripping the handlebars, lie face down on a leg curl machine and place your feet underneath the bar.

Lift:

a. With everything remaining still, raise the bar with your feet by curling your legs as far as you can.

b. Slowly lower your legs towards the starting position the same way you brought them up.

Standing Calf Raises

Prime movers: Calves.

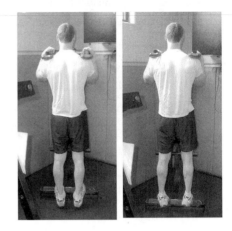

Starting Position: Stand with your shoulders under the supports of a standing calf raise machine and your toes on the elevated stand provided so that your heels are hanging off the end. Keep your back straight and hands gripping the handlebars.

a. With everything remaining still, stand up on your toes as high as you can. Hold the position for a brief moment to maximize the work on your calves.

b. Slowly lower your heels back down towards the starting position the same way you brought them up.

Tip for all calf raises: To ensure the best workout, raise and lower your heels as high and as low as you can, training your calves through the entire range of motion.

Seated Calf Raises

Prime movers: Calves.

Starting Position: Sit with your knees under the supports of a standing calf raise machine and your toes on the elevated stand provided so that your heels are hanging off of the stand. Keep your back straight and hands gripping the handlebars.

a. With everything remaining still, rise up on your toes as high as you can. Hold the position for a brief moment to maximize the work on your calves.

b. Slowly lower your heels back down towards the starting position the same way you brought them up.

Reverse Calf Raises

Prime movers: Front of lower legs.

Starting Position: Stand upright with your heels on an elevated stand or block so that your toes are hanging off the stand. This exercise is best performed with no added resistance other than your body weight.

a. With everything remaining still, stand up on your heels as high as you can. Hold the position for a brief moment to maximize the work on the front of your lower legs.

b. Slowly lower your toes back down towards the starting position the same way you brought them up.

Jump Squats

Prime movers: Upper and lower legs.

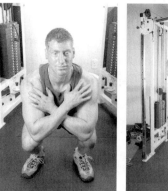
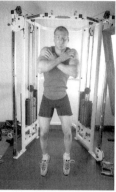

Starting Position: Stand in a squatting position with your feet shoulder-width apart and your arms crossed over your chest. Keep your back straight and your head tilted up.

Lift:

a. With everything remaining still, explosively jump straight up as high as you can.

b. As you land, return to the starting position in one smooth motion.

Power Cleans

Prime movers: Upper and lower legs.

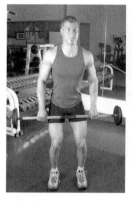
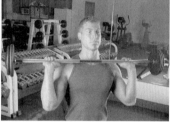

Starting Position: Stand with your back straight and head titled back. Lean slightly forward at the waist so your shoulders are in front of the bar on the floor. Keep your feet at least shoulder-width apart and your knees bent so you can grab a barbell with your arms fully extended, using an overhand grip.

a. Keeping your arms straight, push with your legs and raise the bar up close to your body to your lower thigh with your knees still slightly bent.

b. From this point, use your lower body for momentum to push yourself straight up while simultaneously using your shoulders to raise the bar to your stomach.

c. In one explosive movement, flip your wrists and elbows underneath the bar while simultaneously jumping into a partial squatting position.

Box Steps

Prime movers: Upper and lower legs.

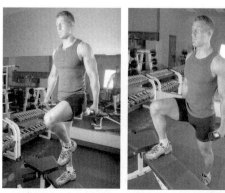

Starting Position: Stand upright with your feet shoulder-width apart and a barbell resting behind your neck on your traps with your hands slightly wider than shoulder-width apart, using an overhand grip or holding dumbbells at your sides. Keep your back straight and your head tilted up. Stand with a box, bench, or some sort of elevated apparatus in front of you.

a. Step forward up on the box or bench with your right foot. Bring your left knee up so that your left thigh is parallel to the floor.

b. Lower your left leg all the way back down to the floor and bring your right leg back down to meet it. Repeat with other leg.

Lunges

Prime movers: Upper and lower legs.

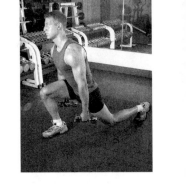

Starting Position: Stand upright with your feet together and either a barbell resting behind your neck on your traps or holding two dumbbells at your sides as in the picture. Your hands should be slightly wider than shoulder-width apart, using an overhand grip. Keep your back straight and your head tilted up.

Lift:

a. With everything remaining still, slowly take a large step forward with one leg, bending both knees. The weight on your back foot should come up on your toes, and the knee on your back leg should come very close, but not touch the floor.

b. Using your extended leg, thrust yourself back to the starting position the same way you came down. The entire lift should be in one smooth, fluid motion.

Tip: The longer your step forward, the more effective this exercise will be.

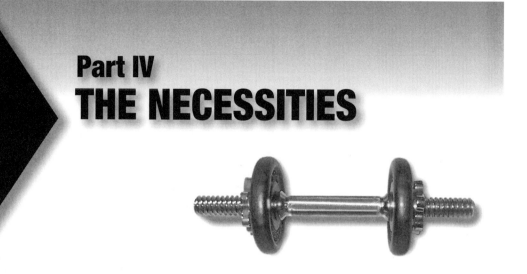

Part IV
THE NECESSITIES

Perfecting Your Technique

This section identifies what you need to accomplish before you begin the program. The information in this section is extremely important for beginners and is also important for experienced weight trainers who have never performed some of the recommended exercises. To follow any type of weight-training routine, you first need to get a feel for the weight room and learn your own strengths.

Now is the time to test out your form, style, and technique. Be sure to take a day or so to perform warm-up sets with each of the exercises listed in that specific program. The object of these first few sessions is not to train so hard that you are sore the following days, but to practice your form and to gain an understanding for yourself and for the weight room. Simply go to the gym with this book, read the recommended exercises section, and go through a few reps of each exercise using very light weights.

These initial days of practice are very important and can be a major help to you as you progress as a weight trainer and athlete by helping you gain an understanding of approximately how much weight you can handle for each exercise.

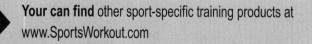

Your can find other sport-specific training products at www.SportsWorkout.com

Estimating Your One Rep Max

 Your one rep max is the greatest amount of weight you can lift one time or for one repetition for a particular exercise.

Knowing your one rep max is an essential part of measuring your strength, your progress, and is very helpful in determining the weight load you should be lifting for every set, regardless of your purpose. This section is called *Estimating* Your One Rep Max because this book never recommends that you *max out*. As discussed in earlier sections, *maxing out* can cause injuries, which, besides being painful and dangerous, can prevent future weight training and baseball or softball. *Auxiliary exercises*, or exercises training smaller muscle groups such as biceps and forearms, can be particularly dangerous when trying to max out. With the estimated one rep max chart provided for you, you can estimate your one rep max without having to attempt to lift your max weight. Instead, you can lift a lighter weight several times to safely and accurately estimate what your max is.

Your estimated one rep max for each exercise is an underlying foundation for weight training. All of the sets and reps you are required to perform are based on percentages of your estimated one rep max.

Understanding the Chart
Steps to finding your estimated one rep max:

1. Choose an exercise that you want to try to find your estimated one rep max.
2. Choose a test weight that is light enough for you to lift several, but not more than, eight times.
3. Lift that weight until failure. If you lift more than eight reps, choose a higher weight and start over.
4. Find your test weight on the far left column of the Estimated One-Rep Max Chart.
5. Find the number of reps you successfully completed on the top row.
6. Scroll right from your test weight and down from your successfully completed reps until you find the number that shares both the same row and column.

The number you arrive at is your estimated one rep max.

For an easier way of determining your one-rep max, log on to **www.sportsworkout.com** to use a **one-rep max calculator.**

REPS

WEIGHT	1	2	3	4	5	6	7	8
5	5	5	5	6	6	6	6	6
10	10	10	11	11	11	12	12	12
15	15	15	16	16	17	17	18	19
20	20	21	21	22	23	23	24	25
25	25	26	27	27	28	29	30	31
30	30	31	32	33	34	35	36	37
35	35	36	37	38	39	41	42	44
40	40	41	42	44	45	47	48	50
45	45	46	48	49	51	52	54	56
50	50	51	53	55	56	58	60	62
55	55	57	58	60	62	64	66	68
60	60	62	64	66	68	70	72	75
65	65	67	69	71	73	76	78	81
70	70	72	74	76	79	81	84	87
75	75	77	79	82	84	87	90	93
80	80	82	85	87	90	93	96	99
85	85	87	90	93	96	99	102	106
90	90	93	95	98	101	105	108	112
95	95	98	101	104	107	110	114	118
100	100	103	106	109	113	116	120	124
105	105	108	111	115	118	122	126	130
110	110	113	117	120	124	128	132	137
115	115	118	122	126	129	134	138	143
120	120	123	127	131	135	139	144	149
125	125	129	132	136	141	145	150	155
130	130	134	138	142	146	151	156	161
135	135	139	143	147	152	157	162	168
140	140	144	148	153	158	163	168	174
145	145	149	154	158	163	168	174	180
150	150	154	159	164	169	174	180	186
155	155	159	164	169	174	180	186	193
160	160	165	169	175	180	186	192	199
165	165	170	175	180	186	192	198	205
170	170	175	180	186	191	197	204	211
175	175	180	185	191	197	203	210	217
180	180	185	191	196	203	209	216	224
185	185	190	196	202	208	215	222	230
190	190	195	201	207	214	221	228	236
195	195	201	207	213	219	227	234	242
200	200	206	212	218	225	232	240	248

REPS

WEIGHT	1	2	3	4	5	6	7	8
205	205	211	217	224	231	238	246	255
210	210	216	222	229	236	244	252	261
215	215	221	228	235	242	250	258	267
220	220	226	233	240	248	256	264	273
225	225	231	238	246	253	261	270	279
230	230	237	244	251	259	267	276	286
235	235	242	249	256	264	273	282	292
240	240	247	254	262	270	279	288	298
245	245	252	259	267	276	285	294	304
250	250	257	265	273	281	290	300	310
255	255	262	270	278	287	296	306	317
260	260	267	275	284	293	302	312	323
265	265	273	281	289	298	308	318	329
270	270	278	286	295	304	314	324	335
275	275	283	291	300	309	319	330	341
280	280	288	297	306	315	325	336	348
285	285	293	302	311	321	331	342	354
290	290	298	307	316	326	337	348	360
295	295	303	312	322	332	343	354	366
300	300	309	318	327	338	348	360	373
305	305	314	323	333	343	354	366	379
310	310	319	328	338	349	360	372	385
315	315	324	334	344	354	366	378	391
320	320	329	339	349	360	372	384	397
325	325	334	344	355	366	378	390	404
330	330	339	349	360	371	383	396	410
335	335	345	355	366	377	389	402	416
340	340	350	360	371	383	395	408	422
345	345	355	365	376	388	401	414	428
350	350	360	371	382	394	407	420	435
355	355	365	376	387	399	412	426	441
360	360	370	381	393	405	418	432	447
365	365	375	387	398	411	424	438	453
370	370	381	392	404	416	430	444	459
375	375	386	397	409	422	436	450	466
380	380	391	402	415	428	441	456	472
385	385	396	408	420	433	447	462	478
390	390	401	413	426	439	453	468	484
395	395	406	418	431	444	459	474	490
400	400	411	424	436	450	465	480	497

REPS

WEIGHT	1	2	3	4	5	6	7	8
405	405	417	429	442	456	470	486	503
410	410	422	434	447	461	476	492	509
415	415	427	439	453	467	482	498	515
420	420	432	445	458	473	488	504	522
425	425	437	450	464	478	494	510	528
430	430	442	455	469	484	499	516	534
435	435	447	461	475	489	505	522	540
440	440	453	466	480	495	511	528	546
445	445	458	471	486	501	517	534	553
450	450	463	477	491	506	523	540	559
455	455	468	482	496	512	529	546	565
460	460	473	487	502	518	534	552	571
465	465	478	492	507	523	540	558	577
470	470	483	498	513	529	546	564	584
475	475	489	503	518	534	552	570	590
480	480	494	508	524	540	558	576	596
485	485	499	514	529	546	563	582	602
490	490	504	519	535	551	569	588	608
495	495	509	524	540	557	575	594	615
500	500	514	529	546	563	581	600	621
505	505	519	535	551	568	587	606	627
510	510	525	540	556	574	592	612	633
515	515	530	545	562	579	598	618	639
520	520	535	551	567	585	604	624	646
525	525	540	556	573	591	610	630	652
530	530	545	561	578	596	616	636	658
535	535	550	567	584	602	621	642	664
540	540	555	572	589	608	627	648	671
545	545	561	577	595	613	633	654	677
550	550	566	582	600	619	639	660	683
555	555	571	588	606	624	645	666	689
560	560	576	593	611	630	650	672	695
565	565	581	598	616	636	656	678	702
570	570	586	604	622	641	662	684	708
575	575	591	609	627	647	668	690	714
580	580	597	614	633	653	674	696	720
585	585	602	619	638	658	679	702	726
590	590	607	625	644	664	685	708	733
595	595	612	630	649	669	691	714	739
600	600	617	635	655	675	697	720	745

The Different Folks, Different Strokes Principle

Like in baseball or softball, in weight training differences between people can occur both physically and mentally. Some people are born with greater muscle-building capabilities than others. A major reason for these genetic differences is the amount of fast-twitch muscle fibers one has. Fast-twitch fibers are able to grow bigger and stronger than the other muscle fibers. Do not feel frustrated if you see others making faster initial gains than you are, because you can and will make enormous gains by following any one of the provided programs. By sticking with your routine and working hard, you can catch and surpass almost everyone. Fast-twitch, as well as slow-twitch fibers, are explained in further detail in the section *Muscle Fibers*.

> **Overtraining** is when you work out so hard that your training negatively affects your goals.

Weight Trainers also differ mentally and psychologically. Different people have different preferences in terms of how they like to work out, what exercises they like to do, as well as how often they like to train. Many of the various programs in this book are based on contrasting styles of equally legitimate training principles. Some programs are for strength and bulk building, others for power enhancement, and still others for increasing endurance, stamina, and burning fat.

Overtraining and Staleness

Everyone, at one point or another, reaches a plateau in his or her training. When this happens, gains are very hard to come by. Many times plateaus occur because of overtraining. Overtraining can occur during one workout, or it can gradually creep up on you over time. It is important to push yourself as hard as you can in the gym and make the most of your time, but there can be a time when you are doing too much. Training seven days a week is an example

> Your muscles need at least forty-eight hours to fully recover from weight training, which is why you should never train the same muscle groups on consecutive days.

of overtraining. We all need rest days so our muscles can recoup, regroup, and rebuild. It is during these days off that your body is able to grow bigger and stronger. Even the best baseball and softball players in the world take at least one day of rest per week.

During one session, some people are able to work out for hours without overtraining, while others simply can't handle that much physical stress. Most beginners will not be able to work out for as long or as often as more experienced weight trainers because their bodies are not yet prepared for that type of strenuous work.

Staleness, on the other hand, is thought by many experts to be a response to overtraining. It is a syndrome that negatively affects your athletic performance and your personality. Rest is the only method of prevention and the only cure for staleness. The program provided for you has been designed so that there is a minimal chance of overtraining and staleness occurring; however, if you do begin to notice symptoms, take at least one week off from weight training and see your physician.

Symptoms of staleness include:

1. Reaching a plateau in training gains
2. Having unusual sleeping patterns
3. Performing tasks seems more difficult
4. Having a decreased appetite leading to unhealthy lean body weight loss
5. Having increased irritability and anxiety
6. Experiencing depression
7. Having a decreased sex drive

Endurance athletes are at the greatest risk of staleness; however, all athletes should be aware of this syndrome regardless of the sport. The different folks, different strokes principle applies to staleness. Many athletes may never experience staleness, but everyone needs to be aware that it can happen.

The Declaration of Variation

Variation is introducing some sort of change in your workout routine. It can be the constant changing of exercises within a program or the compete changing of your program every few weeks. Variation is very important in weight training for several physiological and psychological reasons. Some of the most important benefits of variation in a weight-training program include:

1. **Not allowing your body to adapt to any one routine:** Perhaps the most important reason to vary your routines is so you can keep making progress and gains. Variation is the key to continued progress. Your body is a machine designed to adapt to any stress placed on it, whether it be heat, pressure, or tension. Similarly, your body adapts to the workload you are putting on it in the gym. After following the same routine for long enough, you will plateau because your body has become used to and has adapted to doing the same thing over and over again. When a plateau occurs, you need to shock your body with different types of stimuli to continue making gains. By occasionally switching the type of training you do (how many reps, sets, exercises, and their order), you shock your body so that it has to readapt to the new workload you are putting on it, which enables you to continue to progress.

2. **Keeping you from getting bored:** Following the same routine day after day can become very boring and tiresome. Fitness experts and coaches alike know that boredom in the gym can be a major problem for athletes and other weight trainers. In order to make big gains, you need to train hard and with intensity. Once that intensity is lost, so are the benefits from training hard. When people are bored with their routine, they lose motivation and train with less passion. It is human nature. Unfortunately, this lack of motivation spawns a negative cycle. By not training as hard, gains become more difficult, thus leading to an even greater decrease in motivation, which leads again to not training hard. And so the cycle continues. Varying exercises and styles every so often keeps things fresh and keeps people motivated, especially athletes in the midst of a long off-season.

3. Targeting, strengthening, and toning every part of every muscle: As you've noticed, this book provides you with many weight-training exercises. Many of these exercises train the same muscle groups. Like people, no two exercises are exactly alike. Some may be similar, but not identical. Each exercise targets your muscle from a different angle and achieves a different benefit. By using a variety of exercises on the same muscles, you strengthen every part of those muscles.

Muscle Fibers
(How to Train, What and Why)

Our muscles are made up of many bundles of muscle fibers. Each fiber type has its own characteristics and purposes. For simplicity purposes, these muscle fibers can be categorized as:

1. **Fast-Twitch Fibers**
2. **Slow-Twitch Fibers**
3. **Intermediate Fibers (properties of both)**

The muscle-fiber makeup in most people is roughly 25% fast twitch, 25% slow twitch, and 50% intermediate fibers, which contain properties of both fast- and slow-twitch muscle fibers. With proper training some of the intermediate fibers can be converted to fast- or slow–twitch fibers. The more fast-twitch fibers one has, the more powerful and explosive he or she will be. People with more slow-twitch fibers will have greater endurance and stamina. Depending on your purpose, you can weight train in order to build up either muscle fiber.

Fast-Twitch Fibers

Generally, fast-twitch fibers are used in strength and explosive sports or sports that require bursts of speed and power for relatively short amounts of time. A running back bursting through a hole, a baseball or softball player trying to beat out an infield hit, a basketball player exploding up to the hoop for a slam, a golfer ripping a drive three hundred yards off the tee, a tennis player smashing a backhand across the court, a short distance swimmer torpedoing through the water, and a 110 hurdler flying down the lane are all putting their fast-twitch fibers to the test. Any type of explosive movement is being performed by fast-twitch fibers. People who participate in these or similar types of activities should concentrate primarily on working their fast-twitch fibers

The simple reason more fast-twitch muscle fibers lead to better performance in explosive activities is because they contract faster and with more power than slow-twitch fibers. Fast-twitch fibers lead to *hypertrophy*—an increase in the size of muscle fibers as an outcome of weight training—more easily than slow-twitch fibers. As your muscle fibers increase in size, so do your muscles. The downside to fast-twitch fibers is that they can only work at full capacity for short periods of time before fatiguing because they work primarily without oxygen, or *anaerobically*, and get most of their energy from limited stores of muscle glycogen.

Slow-Twitch Fibers

Slow-twitch fibers are used in stamina and endurance-based activities. Long distance runners, cyclists, swimmers, and triathletes are examples of people who should concentrate on slow-twitch training. Slow-twitch fibers contract more slowly than fast-twitch fibers, but are able to work for hours longer if trained properly. Slow-twitch fibers get their energy aerobically, from oxygen. Slow-twitch training is great for burning fat because oxygen stimulates the use of fat for energy. There is less hypertrophy in slow-twitch fibers, which is why marathon runners tend to be much smaller than football players.

Training Techniques

Training to Failure: Training to failure means training in a particular set until you exhaust yourself and cannot complete another repetition on your own. Whether you are training for endurance, power, or strength, it is recommended that you train to failure in most of your sets. By training to failure, you train your body to its maximum capabilities. This type of training is tough, but well worth the results.

Forced Reps: Forced reps are performed directly after you have trained to positive failure and cannot complete another repetition. You lower the weight regularly and your partner helps you slowly lift it back up. Your partner should assist you to complete the rep, but not do all of the work for you. Your partner should make sure you spend at least three or four seconds on the positive phase of the lift while assisting you.

Negatives: Negatives are also performed directly after you have trained to failure. The opposite of forced reps, the eccentric, or lowering aspect of the lift, is extremely slow, and the concentric part of the lift is fast, with the help of your partner. It should take you approximately six or seven seconds to lower the weights with the help of your partner. At this point, with the help from a spotter, quickly return the weights to their starting position and repeat. Using negatives is the best method for increasing strength and size; however, they should not be used very often because they work your muscles so hard they need over a week in order to fully recover before performing them again.

Supersets: This is a training method where you perform one set of two exercises sequentially without rest. For example, if you were to superset preacher curls with triceps curls, you would do one set of preachers and immediately after completion, do one set of triceps curls and then rest before repeating.

> You are able to perform negatives with weights higher than your one rep max because eccentrically you can lift a great deal more than you can concentrically.

Tri Sets: Same as Supersets but with three exercises instead of two.

Pre-exhaust: This method is one of the most intense methods of weight training. It is a form of supersetting where you perform many reps of a single-joint exercise and immediately follow it up with a compound exercise training the same muscles. For example, if you were to pre-exhaust your shoulders, you would first perform many reps of light lateral raises and immediately follow it up with a military press.

Burnouts (stripping method): This method is very popular and very effective. Directly after you complete a set working to failure, immediately lighten the load of the weights so you can continue to train without rest, and perform the next set to failure where you will again lighten the load and work to failure.

Pyramid Method: The pyramid method is a great strength-building tactic. It is performed properly by decreasing the reps and increasing the weight with every set. An example would be performing five reps with 100 lbs. followed by three reps with 120 lbs. and one rep with 140 lbs.

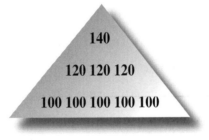

21's: This method is most often performed for biceps exercises, particularly for preacher curls. These exercises are properly executed by performing seven reps going from the bottom of the lift to the halfway point and back for seven reps, then performing seven reps going from the halfway point to the top, followed by seven reps through the complete range of motion.

Cycling: Cycling is rotating between two or three different routines. As long as the routines are different, it is considered cycling. A holistic cycle would be following an endurance program, then a power program, and then a strength program. It is best to take one week of active or complete rest after you have completed a full cycle to let your body completely recover before beginning again. Active rest is any sort of low-level, non-structured activity.

Circuit Training: Circuit training is the best method of weight training for total fitness and aerobic benefits. It is a great way to get a fast and effective full-body workout. Circuit training is a type of endurance training in which you perform one set of six to ten exercises consecutively without rest. The six to ten exercises should train the major muscle groups of your entire body for a complete workout. After you have completed one circuit through the entire rotation, rest for a short time before repeating.

When to Increase
(The X + 3 Method)

> **Rule of thumb:** Increase the number of reps before increasing the weight.

The goal of weight training is to gradually increase the resistance over time. Two ways of increasing the resistance are:

1. **Increasing the weight**
2. **Increasing the number of reps**

Increasing the weight you lift can be overwhelming and difficult, so this book recommends that once a weight begins to feel too light for the designated number of repetitions, increase the number of reps before increasing the weight. The X + 3 method states that if you are required to lift X reps in a given set and are able to accomplish it, then the next time you lift, go for X + 1 reps using the same weight. As each exercise begins to feel lighter and lighter, increase your reps up until X + 3. When reps of X + 3 become easily attainable, increase the weight by 5 lbs. and return to reps of X, repeating this entire process. While training smaller, auxiliary-muscle groups like your biceps, triceps and forearms, make increases by 2 pounds at a time. Below is an example of the X + 3 method.

Your routine requires you to bench 100 lbs. 10 times. You complete the 10 reps with ease and the next time you go to the gym you lifts 100 lbs. 11 times. You continue this process until benching 100 lbs. 13 times becomes easy. At this point, you increase your bench to 105 lbs. and start back with 10 reps.

Choosing the Right Program

Provided for you are 54 programs/routines. Each one is designed for a different purpose. How do you know which one to choose? Below are important factors to consider when selecting your program:

Purpose: The most important factor to consider when choosing your program is the purpose for which you are training. Do you want to get bigger, stronger, more toned, more powerful, leaner, or do you want to train for general fitness? If you want to get big and choose an endurance program, you will be working away from your goal. Make sure you choose a program that fits your purpose.

Weight-Training Experience: The second factor to consider while choosing your program is your experience in the gym. For each style of training, you are offered different levels of intensity. If you are a beginner, you probably want to start out with a program of less time and frequency than the more advanced programs provided so you do not run the risk of overtraining. Likewise, if you are experienced in weight training and are looking to take the next step, you will most likely follow a program with more exercises and greater frequency to get a better workout.

Time Availability: Your time availability is also a major factor in determining your program. You are provided with programs ranging from three to six days per week. For each style, you can choose between six levels of difficulty based on the amount of exercises and the frequency of your training. If you do not have much time to train, then choose a Level I or Level II program. If you have a lot of time to train and have the desire to train hard, then choose a Level IV or Level V program. Level VI programs are recommended only for the very advanced weight trainers. Assuming you train with the same intensity, you will see results faster by training with a more difficult program.

Personal Preference: This is the final element you should use while determining your program. The next section explains your choices.

Personal Preference

Once you have found all of the programs that meet your criteria in terms of purpose, experience, and time availability, you can make your final decision based on your personal preference. Take a look at each of the programs and decide which style of training you like more. You can choose between training *antagonistic* (opposite) muscle groups or *synergistic* (goal-congruent) muscle groups on the same day. These are the two major styles of weight training. Both are excellent ways of working out and are used equally by numerous athletes, body builders, and weight lifters. The styles are:

Antagonistic (Opposite) Muscle Training

Pros: By training antagonistic muscle groups on the same day, you are stretching your muscles and increasing your flexibility and range of motion. For example, while training your triceps, you are extending your arm, which stretches your biceps. You can become very flexible by using this style of training and stretching during your cooling down period.

Examples of antagonistic-muscle groups include:
Biceps/Triceps
Chest/Lats (Back)
Hamstrings/Quadriceps (thighs)
Abdominals/Lower Back

Cons: The major problem that arises from this style of training is fatigue. The larger the muscle group you are training, the more fatigued you will become. When training antagonistic muscle groups, you will train your chest and your lats (back) on the same day. These are both very large muscle groups, and, if you are training hard, you may experience some fatigue.

> The larger the muscle group you are training, the more fatigued you will become.

Synergistic (Goal-Congruent) Muscle Training: "The Push-Pull Method"

Pros: Training synergistically allows you to train your muscles with even greater focus because every exercise you perform will be training at least one common muscle. Examples of synergistic training include training your chest and triceps on the same day because they both work out the triceps. Another example of this is working your lats (back) and your biceps, both training your biceps. This type of training is referred to as the *push-pull method* because you will be performing all of your pushing exercises on one day and all of your pulling exercises on the next.

Cons: The only true cost of training this way is that you do not get the stretch in your muscles during your weight-training session as you do in opposite-muscle training. If your sport requires serious flexibility, you may be better off training with the antagonistic muscle approach.

> It is best if you periodically switch from one style to the next to shock your body with a different type of training. Try out both of the major styles of training and determine for yourself what works best for you.

Program Levels

All of the programs are broken down into six levels of difficulty. The least intense programs are Level I for beginners or for people without much time to spend in the gym. The most intense programs are Level VI, which are to be used exclusively by experienced weight trainers looking to take their training to the next stage. The Level I programs have been created to be easier on your body while still allowing you to make progress, and the Level VI programs have been created to train you as hard as possible without overtraining. The more intense the program, the faster you will see results.

Level I: Beginners

Level II: Somewhat intense

Level III: Moderate intensity

Level IV: Above average intensity

Level V: Very intense

Level VI: Extremely Intense — Recommended only for experienced weight trainers.

The program levels are not based on how hard you train while in the gym. The levels are based on three other factors:

1. **Frequency**
2. **Time**
3. **Advanced training methods**

Frequency: The programs provided for you are either three or four days per week, allowing you to increase them up to six days per week—except strength-training programs, which must not exceed five days per week. Therefore, the more frequent the program has you working out, the greater the total intensity of the program.

Three-days–a-week programs: Our least frequent programs require you to train three days per week. Anything less would not be enough training for you to make gains. Training twice a week is considered to be *maintenance training*, allowing you to do nothing more than maintain the gains you have already made.

Each one of the three-days-a-week programs trains your entire body in one session and can be performed by circuit training if you desire. Circuit training is explained in more detail in *Training Techniques*. Because you are training your entire body in one session, you are not able to put much focus on any one muscle group. Training a minimum of three days a week ensures that you are working every muscle in your body the required number of times per week to continue making gains. Also, because you are training your entire body during one session, the following day is always a rest day, providing your muscles with sufficient time to recoup and regroup.

Four plus days a week programs: As the frequency of the program grows, so do the choices. When you train more than three days per week, you cannot train your entire body in one single day because you would not be able to take a day of rest after every training session. With these more frequent programs, you can choose whether you want to follow a two- or three-day split. Training different muscle groups each day gives your muscles time to rest while other muscles are being trained, enabling you to train in consecutive days. Notice that you are never required to train all seven days of the week because your body needs at least one full day of rest to heal and grow stronger.

If you choose to increase the frequency of your prescribed program, bump up its level of difficulty by one.

Time: Certain programs contain more exercises than others. The number of required exercises relates directly to the time you will be spending in the gym. The more exercises the program has, the higher the intensity level will be.

Advanced-training methods: The last factor determining the level of the program is the use of advanced-training methods. These methods include negatives, supersets, forced reps, pre-exhausts, and burnouts, which are explained in further detail in the next section.

Advanced-training methods are optional throughout each program. The use of advanced training methods moves the difficulty of the program up one level.

Each of the programs is designed for you to make serious gains and positive changes to your body, mind, health, and athletic ability. The more intense the program, the quicker you will be able to achieve and surpass your goals. The harder you train, the faster your muscles will respond. These programs have been carefully created so that you do not over- or undertrain yourself based on principles regarding sufficient time to rest and train your muscles.

Safety Reminders

When done properly, weight training can be a very effective way to sculpt your body and achieve your athletic potential. On top of all of the performance-enhancing benefits to weight training, it also plays a major role in injury reduction, injury prevention, and injury rehabilitation. With stronger muscles supporting your bones, tendons, and ligaments, you will be much less injury prone and will able to perform most activities hard and strong all the time. However, if necessary safety precautions are not followed, injuries can result.

Listed below are a few safety reminders to help keep you injury free in the gym.

Always use a spotter: It does not matter how experienced you are or how light you think the weight is, you always need someone to spot you.

Use safety collars: Collars will prevent weights from tipping over during a lift, which can result in an injury to you or others.

Pick up weights properly: Most injuries in the weight room come from picking up and putting weights down improperly. To avoid chronic lower-back problems, be sure to bend at the knees and to keep your back straight every time you pick up or put down weights.

Drink enough water: Even if you are not thirsty, be sure to drink lots of water before and during your workout, especially if you anticipate a lot of perspiration. As you become dehydrated, your ability to perform work drops way off, which will limit your intensity and slow your progress.

Use proper form: Proper form will provide you with the best results and help keep you injury free.

Breathe correctly: It is very important to simply breathe while performing any exercise, inhaling on the negative part of the lift and exhaling on the positive part. Do not hold your breath! .

Do not drop weights: Not only can this break the weights, but it can also be very dangerous for everyone in the gym. Always put the weights back in a controlled manner.

Dress properly: Gym shoes are a must; wearing inappropriate gym attire like sandals can results in injuries such as broken toes.

Use your head: If you begin to feel sick, queasy, light-headed, or if you experience joint or chest pains, stop your session and get yourself checked out immediately.

Consult your physician: It is required for everyone to check with his or her physician before beginning any one of the prescribed programs or before increasing the intensity to any of the programs.

Record Keeping

When following any type of program, it is vital that you keep daily records for many reasons. Five of the most important are:

1. **Knowing when to increase the weight or reps**
2. **Knowing where to start after taking time away from the gym**
3. **Observing your gains over time**
4. **Motivation**
5. **Detect overtraining**

You can keep records on any or all of a vast number of factors that may be important to your training or progress. You have been provided with an example of a record-keeping chart to help you monitor your progress. You can print an unlimited amount of these charts from **www.sportsworkout.com/chart.htm.** They have been made accessible so you can keep records in the very best and easiest way possible. To complement the record-keeping chart, there is a *testing sheet*, which can also be printed from the Web site at **www.sportsworkout.com/test.htm.** With the testing sheets, you will be able to use formulas to literally put your strength, power, endurance, and athletic ability to the test.

> You can find well-designed printable record-keeping charts at **www.sportsworkout.com/chart.htm** that are designed to work with any one of the provided routines, and testing sheets at **www.sportsworkout.com/test.htm** where you can test your progress in many fashions.

When to increase: Keeping records of your daily activity in the gym will allow you to determine when you are ready to increase the workload and by how much. Without well-kept records, your attempts to intensify your weight-training regimen will be made with hit or miss tactics. These tactics are not efficient ways to make gains because you will waste time by approximating your weight-loads and you may not be pushing yourself hard enough with the proper resistance. With well-kept records, you will know exactly when you need to increase the load and by how much.

Where to start: At one point or another, there will be instances when you will be unable to make it to the gym for extended periods of time. It may be because you become ill, experience a death in the family, or go on a vacation. The bottom line is there may be a time when you will stop your program and need to re-enter it. By keeping records, you will know exactly where you left off. Because you have taken time away from lifting, however, you will need to slightly decrease the load from where you left off, but you will have your records as a measuring stick. This is a very important aspect to training. If you take an extended period of time away from lifting without maintaining records, you will have to go by memory, which will result in trial and error once again.

Observe your gains: It is very important to be able to observe your gains for several reasons. The most important is that with well-kept records, you will be able to see which parts of the body you have made improvements in and which parts still need work. The records give you a sense of what changes need to be made for your next program to make up for these differences. You will want to saturate your next program with more exercises that train the weaker areas of your body, and this information can only be known with well-kept records.

Motivation: On top of monitoring your progress in the gym, record keeping provides you with the motivation to continue working harder and making bigger gains. You will literally be able to see on paper how you have progressed over time, which will inspire you to want to train harder. When people have hard evidence that they are actually making gains in the gym, it motivates them to continue making those gains.

Overtraining: How are record keeping and overtraining related? Even if you do not feel overtrained, you will be able to clearly see if you are overtrained by looking at your records. If, over time, you notice decreases from one day to the next in your records, the culprit may be overtraining. Overtraining may not always be the reason, but it very well could be. Other reasons could be changes in your eating or sleeping pattern or illness. In any case, record keeping will help you determine what the problem may be and how you can fix it.

Top Left Chart

DATE:		BODY WT:	Hours of Sleep:				
Time IN:	Time OUT:	Other:					
		Set 1	Set 2	Set 3	Set 4	Set 5	

Larger printable record keeping charts can be found at www.sportsworkout.com/chart.htm

EXERCISE:	WEIGHT					
	DESIRED REPS					
	COMPLETED REPS					
EXERCISE:	WEIGHT					
	DESIRED REPS					
	COMPLETED REPS					
EXERCISE:	WEIGHT					
	DESIRED REPS					
	COMPLETED REPS					
EXERCISE:	WEIGHT					
	DESIRED REPS					
	COMPLETED REPS					
EXERCISE:	WEIGHT					
	DESIRED REPS					
	COMPLETED REPS					
EXERCISE:	WEIGHT					
	DESIRED REPS					
	COMPLETED REPS					
EXERCISE:	WEIGHT					
	DESIRED REPS					
	COMPLETED REPS					
EXERCISE:	WEIGHT					
	DESIRED REPS					
	COMPLETED REPS					

Top Right Chart

DATE:		BODY WT:	Hours of Sleep:				
Time IN:	Time OUT:	Other:					
		Set 1	Set 2	Set 3	Set 4	Set 5	

EXERCISE:	WEIGHT					
	DESIRED REPS					
	COMPLETED REPS					
EXERCISE:	WEIGHT					
	DESIRED REPS					
	COMPLETED REPS					
EXERCISE:	WEIGHT					
	DESIRED REPS					
	COMPLETED REPS					
EXERCISE:	WEIGHT					
	DESIRED REPS					
	COMPLETED REPS					
EXERCISE:	WEIGHT					
	DESIRED REPS					
	COMPLETED REPS					
EXERCISE:	WEIGHT					
	DESIRED REPS					
	COMPLETED REPS					
EXERCISE:	WEIGHT					
	DESIRED REPS					
	COMPLETED REPS					

Bottom Left Chart

DATE:		BODY WT:	Hours of Sleep:				
Time IN:	Time OUT:	Other:					
		Set 1	Set 2	Set 3	Set 4	Set 5	

EXERCISE:	WEIGHT					
	DESIRED REPS					
	COMPLETED REPS					
EXERCISE:	WEIGHT					
	DESIRED REPS					
	COMPLETED REPS					
EXERCISE:	WEIGHT					
	DESIRED REPS					
	COMPLETED REPS					
EXERCISE:	WEIGHT					
	DESIRED REPS					
	COMPLETED REPS					
EXERCISE:	WEIGHT					
	DESIRED REPS					
	COMPLETED REPS					
EXERCISE:	WEIGHT					
	DESIRED REPS					
	COMPLETED REPS					
EXERCISE:	WEIGHT					
	DESIRED REPS					
	COMPLETED REPS					
EXERCISE:	WEIGHT					
	DESIRED REPS					
	COMPLETED REPS					

Bottom Right Chart

DATE:		BODY WT:	Hours of Sleep:				
Time IN:	Time OUT:	Other:					
		Set 1	Set 2	Set 3	Set 4	Set 5	

EXERCISE:	WEIGHT					
	DESIRED REPS					
	COMPLETED REPS					
EXERCISE:	WEIGHT					
	DESIRED REPS					
	COMPLETED REPS					
EXERCISE:	WEIGHT					
	DESIRED REPS					
	COMPLETED REPS					
EXERCISE:	WEIGHT					
	DESIRED REPS					
	COMPLETED REPS					
EXERCISE:	WEIGHT					
	DESIRED REPS					
	COMPLETED REPS					
EXERCISE:	WEIGHT					
	DESIRED REPS					
	COMPLETED REPS					
EXERCISE:	WEIGHT					
	DESIRED REPS					
	COMPLETED REPS					
EXERCISE:	WEIGHT					
	DESIRED REPS					
	COMPLETED REPS					

Test Yourself!

By testing yourself, you can visually see the gains you have made, and how extensive they have been. Provided for you at **www.sportsworkout.com/test.htm** are strength, power, endurance, and sport-specific tests so you can measure your progress in every fashion. You can also keep track of other important variables such as body weight, as well as muscle and waistline measurements.

Retest yourself every six weeks to monitor your gains.

You can apply the strength, power, or endurance tests to any and all of the recommended exercises. However, it is suggested that you only test yourself in the bench press, leg press, military press, and lat pull because it would take days for you to test yourself in each of the recommended exercises. These four exercises are good indications of your overall fitness because they cover all of your major muscle groups. The bench press works your chest and triceps. The leg press covers your entire lower body. The lat pull has you working your lats and biceps. And military press trains your shoulders and traps.

The website provides you with several ways of testing yourself so that you will know exactly what you have improved in and what you may still need work on. For every non-weight-training related test, take the best of three tests to ensure the most accurate results.

Conclusion

You are now ready to begin weight training for baseball or softball. You have all of the information in front of you and expert-designed programs for your use, equipping you with the best methods available to improve your athletic potential. You also know how to apply the exercises properly. With hard work and determination, you will achieve any goals you set for yourself. Best of luck training and best of luck on the diamond.

To continue to maximize your training, be sure to check out other baseball or softball-related training books and products at **www.sportsworkout.com**.

Part V
THE PROGRAMS

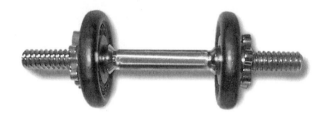

Endurance/Fat Burning Training

Program Level I
Endurance/Fat Burning Training
Entire body every training day
Rest every other day

Weeks 1 and 2

Day 1

exercise	sets	reps
barbell bench press	3	20
seated cable rows	3	20
squats	3	20
dumbbell military press	3	20

Day 2

exercise	sets	reps
incline barbell bench press	3	20
one arm dumbbell rows	3	20
leg press	3	20
barbell military press	3	20

Day 3

exercise	sets	reps
barbell bench press	3	20
seated cable rows	3	20
squats	3	20
dumbbell military press	3	20

Weeks 3 and 4

Day 1

exercise	sets	reps
barbell bench press	3	25
seated cable rows	3	25
squats	3	25
dumbbell military press	3	25

Day 2

exercise	sets	reps
incline barbell bench press	3	25
one arm dumbbell rows	3	25
leg press	3	25
barbell military press	3	25

Day 3

exercise	sets	reps
barbell bench press	3	25
seated cable rows	3	25
squats	3	25
dumbbell military press	3	25

Program Level II
Endurance/Fat Burning Training
Entire body every training day
Rest every other day

Weeks 1 and 2

Day 1

exercise	sets	reps
barbell bench press	3	20
seated cable rows	3	20
squats	3	20
dumbbell military press	3	20
lunges	3	20
front raises	2	20

Day 2

exercise	sets	reps
dumbbell bench press	3	20
standing flyes	3	20
bent-over barbell rows	3	20
leg curls	3	20
standing calf raises	3	20
cable crossovers	2	20

Day 3

exercise	sets	reps
barbell bench press	3	20
seated cable rows	3	20
squats	3	20
dumbbell military press	3	20
lunges	3	20

Weeks 3 and 4

Day 1

exercise	sets	reps
barbell bench press	3	25
seated cable rows	3	25
squats	3	25
dumbbell military press	3	25
lunges	3	25

Day 2

exercise	sets	reps
dumbbell bench press	3	25
standing flyes	3	25
bent-over barbell rows	3	25
leg curls	3	25
standing calf raises	3	25

Day 3

exercise	sets	reps
barbell bench press	3	25
seated cable rows	3	25
squats	3	25
dumbbell military press	3	25
lunges	3	25
front raises	2	25

Program Level II
Endurance/Fat Burning Training
Three-Day Split four days a week
Antagonistic Training

Weeks 1 and 2

Day 1

exercise	sets	reps
barbell bench press	3	20
dumbbell incline bench press	2	20
seated cable rows	3	20

Day 2

exercise	sets	reps
triceps kickbacks	2	20
bench dips	2	20
dumbbell curls	2	20
incline curls	2	20

Day 3

exercise	sets	reps
squats	3	20
leg curls	2	20
dumbbell military press	3	20
upright rows	3	20

Weeks 3 and 4

Day 1

exercise	sets	reps
dumbbell bench press	3	25
incline barbell bench press	2	25
one-arm dumbbell rows	3	25
T-bar rows	2	25

Day 2

exercise	sets	reps
preacher curls	2	25
reverse curls	2	25
barbell triceps curls	2	25
bench dips	2	25

Day 3

exercise	sets	reps
leg press	3	25
lunges	3	25
barbell military press	3	25
front raises	2	25

Program Level II
Endurance/Fat Burning Training
Three-Day Split four days a week
Synergistic Training

Weeks 1 and 2

Day 1

exercise	sets	reps
dumbbell bench press	3	20
incline barbell bench press	3	20
triceps kickbacks	2	20
bench dips	2	failure

Day 2

exercise	sets	reps
seated cable rows	3	20
bent-over barbell rows	3	20
dumbbell curls	2	20
incline curls	2	20

Day 3

exercise	sets	reps
squats	3	20
leg extensions	2	20
dumbbell military press	3	20

Weeks 3 and 4

Day 1

exercise	sets	reps
barbell bench press	3	25
dumbbell incline bench press	3	25
triceps curls	3	25

Day 2

exercise	sets	reps
one-arm rows	3	25
T-bar rows	3	25
preacher curls	2	25
barbell curls	2	25

Day 3

exercise	sets	reps
leg press	3	25
lunges	3	25
barbell military press	3	25
front raises	2	25

Program Level III
Endurance/Fat Burning Training
Three-Day Split four days a week--Antagonistic Training

Weeks 1 and 2

Day 1

exercise	sets	reps
barbell bench press	3	20
dumbbell incline bench press	2	20
seated cable rows	3	20
bent-over barbell rows	2	20
dips	3	failure
wide-grip lat pull downs	2	20

Day 2

exercise	sets	reps
triceps kickbacks	2	20
bench dips	2	20
dumbbell curls	2	20
incline curls	2	20
hammer curls	2	20
close-grip bench press	2	20

Day 3

exercise	sets	reps
squats	3	20
leg extensions	2	20
dumbbell military press	3	20
upright rows	3	20
lunges	2	20

Weeks 3 and 4

Day 1

exercise	sets	reps
dumbbell bench press	3	25
incline barbell bench press	2	25
one-arm dumbbell rows	3	25
T-bar rows	2	25
cable crossovers	2	25
close-grip lat pull downs	2	25

Day 2

exercise	sets	reps
preacher curls	2	25
reverse curls	2	25
dumbbell triceps curls	2	25
bench dips	2	25
triceps pull downs	2	25
barbell curls	2	25

Day 3

exercise	sets	reps
leg press	3	25
lunges	3	25
barbell Military press	3	25
lateral raises	2	25
seated calf raises	3	25

Program Level III
Endurance/Fat Burning Training
Three-Day Split four days a week--Synergistic Training

Weeks 1 and 2

Day 1

exercise	sets	reps
dumbbell bench press	3	20
incline barbell bench press	3	20
triceps kickbacks	2	20
bench dips	2	failure
close-grip bench press	2	20
dips	3	failure

Day 2

exercise	sets	reps
seated cable rows	3	20
bent-over barbell rows	3	20
dumbbell curls	2	20
incline curls	2	20
wide-grip lat pull downs	3	20

Day 3

exercise	sets	reps
squats	3	20
leg curls	2	20
dumbbell military press	3	20
upright rows	3	20
lunges	2	20

Weeks 3 and 4

Day 1

exercise	sets	reps
barbell bench press	3	25
incline dumbbell bench press	3	25
triceps curls	3	25
bench dips	2	failure
cable crossovers	2	25

Day 2

exercise	sets	reps
one-arm dumbbell rows	3	25
T- bar rows	3	25
preacher curls	2	25
barbell curls	2	25
close-grip lat pull downs	3	25
concentration curls	2	25

Day 3

exercise	sets	reps
leg press	3	25
lunges	3	25
barbell military press	3	25
lateral raises	2	25
seated calf raises	3	25

Program Level III
Endurance/Fat Burning Training
Two-Day Split 4 days per week
Upper & lower body training on the same day
Antagonistic Training

Weeks 1 and 2

Days 1 and 3

exercise	sets	reps
barbell bench press	3	20
dumbbell military press	3	20
wide-grip pull-ups	3	20
leg press	3	20

Days 2 and 4

exercise	sets	reps
leg curls	3	20
standing calf raises	3	20
dumbbell curls	2	20

Weeks 3 and 4

Days 1 and 3

exercise	sets	reps
dumbbell bench press	3	25
barbell military press	3	25
close-grip lat pull downs	3	25
leg curls	2	25

Days 2 and 4

exercise	sets	reps
squats	3	25
seated calf raises	2	25
barbell curls	2	25
one-arm triceps extension	2	25

Program Level III
Endurance/Fat Burning Training
Two-Day Split 4 days per week
Upper & lower body training on different days

Weeks 1 and 2

Days 1 and 3

exercise	sets	reps
barbell bench press	3	20,20,20
barbell military press	3	20,20,20
bent-over dumbbell rows	3	20,20,20
hammer curls	2	20,20

Days 2 and 4

exercise	sets	reps
squats	3	20,20,20
leg press	3	20,20,20
seated calf raises	3	20,20,20
lunges	2	20,20

Weeks 3 and 4

Days 1 and 3

exercise	sets	reps
dumbbell bench press	3	25,25,25
dumbbell military press	3	25,25,25
bent-over barbell rows	3	25,25,25
reverse dumbbell curls	2	25,25

Days 2 and 4

exercise	sets	reps
leg press	3	20,20,20
lunges	2	20,20,20
squats	3	20,20,20
standing calf raises	3	20,20

Program Level III
Endurance/Fat Burning Training
Two-Day Split 4 days per week
Upper & lower body training on the same day -- Synergistic Training

Weeks 1 and 2

Days 1 and 3

exercise	sets	reps
barbell bench press	3	20
dumbbell incline bench press	2	20
standing flyes	3	20
leg press	3	20

Days 2 and 4

exercise	sets	reps
wide-grip pull-ups	2	failure
hammer curls	2	20
leg curls	3	20
standing calf raises	3	20

Weeks 3 and 4

Days 1 and 3

exercise	sets	reps
dumbbell bench press	3	25
barbell incline bench press	2	25
upright rows	3	25
squats	3	25

Days 2 and 4

exercise	sets	reps
close-grip pull-ups	2	failure
reverse curls	2	25
leg curls	3	25
seated calf raises	2	25

Program Level III
Endurance/Fat Burning Training
Entire body every training day -- Rest every other day

Weeks 1 and 2

Day 1

exercise	sets	reps
barbell bench press	3	20
seated cable rows	3	20
squats	3	20
dumbbell military press	3	20
lunges	3	20
front raises	2	20
incline flyes	2	20

Day 2

exercise	sets	reps
dumbbell bench press	3	20
standing flyes	3	20
bent-over barbell rows	3	20
leg curls	3	20
standing calf raises	3	20
cable crossovers	2	20
barbell military press	2	20

Day 3

exercise	sets	reps
bench	3	20
seated cable rows	3	20
squats	3	20
dumbbell military	3	20
lunges	3	20
front raises	2	20
incline flys	2	20

Weeks 3 and 4

Day 1

exercise	sets	reps
barbell bench press	3	25
seated cable rows	3	25
squats	3	25
dumbbell military press	3	25
lunges	3	25
front raises	2	25
incline flyes	2	25

Day 2

exercise	sets	reps
dumbbell bench press	3	25
standing flyes	3	25
bent-over barbell rows	3	25
leg curls	3	25
standing calf raises	3	25
cable crossovers	2	25
barbell military press	2	25

Day 3

exercise	sets	reps
barbell bench press	3	25
seated cable rows	3	25
squats	3	25
dumbbell military press	3	25
lunges	3	25
front raises	2	25
incline flyes	2	25

Program Level IV
Endurance/Fat Burning Training
Three-Day Split four days a week -- Antagonistic Training

Weeks 1 and 2

Day 1

exercise	sets	reps
barbell bench press	3	20
dumbbell incline bench press	2	20
seated cable rows	3	20
bent-over barbell rows	2	20
dips	3	failure
wide-grip lat pull downs	2	20
flyes	2	20

Day 2

exercise	sets	reps
triceps kickbacks	2	20
bench dips	2	20
dumbbell curls	2	20
incline curls	2	20
hammer curls	2	20
close-grip bench press	2	20
triceps push downs	2	20

Day 3

exercise	sets	reps
squats	3	20
leg curls	2	20
dumbbell military press	3	20
upright rows	3	20
lunges	2	20
bent-over lateral raises	2	20
standing flyes	2	20

Weeks 3 and 4

Day 1

exercise	sets	reps
dumbbell bench press	3	25
incline barbell bench press	2	25
one-arm dumbbell rows	3	25
T-bar rows	2	25
cable crossovers	2	25
close-grip lat pull downs	2	25
dips	3	failure

Day 2

exercise	sets	reps
preacher curls	2	25
reverse curls	2	25
barbell triceps curls	2	25
bench dips	2	25
triceps pull downs	2	25
barbell curls	2	25
reverse wrist curls	2	25

Day 3

exercise	sets	reps
leg press	3	25
lunges	3	25
barbell military press	3	25
lateral raises	2	25
seated calf raises	3	25
cable lateral raises	2	25
dumbbell shrugs	3	25

www.sportsworkout.com

Program Level IV
Endurance/Fat Burning Training
Three-Day Split four days a week -- Synergistic Training

Weeks 1 and 2

Day 1

exercise	sets	reps
barbell bench press	3	10,10,10
dumbbell incline bench press	3	12,12,12
bench dips	3	failure
dumbbells triceps curls	3	15,15,15
cable crossovers	3	15,15,15
one-arm triceps extensions	3	15,15,15
dips	3	failure

Day 2

exercise	sets	reps
wide-grip lat pull down	3	10,10,10
T-bar row	3	12,12,12
barbell curls	3	failure
concentration curls	3	15,15,15
seated cable rows	3	15,15,15
bent-over barbell rows	3	15,15,15
hammer curls	3	12,12,12

Day 3

exercise	sets	reps
jump squats	3	10,10,10
power cleans	3	12,12,12
dumbbell military press	3	10,10,10
push press	3	12,12,12
leg press	3	8,8,8
bent-over lateral raises	3	15,15,15
standing flyes	3	12,12,12

Weeks 3 and 4

Day 1

exercise	sets	reps
dumbbell bench press	3	10,10,10
incline barbell bench press	3	12,12,12
close-grip bench press	3	12,12,12
skull crushers	3	15,15,15
incline flyes	3	15,15,15
triceps push downs	3	15,15,15
dips	3	failure

Day 2

exercise	sets	reps
close-grip pull-ups	3	failure
seated cable rows	3	10,10,10
preacher curls	3	15,15,15
concentration curls	3	15,15,15
bent-over dumbbell rows	3	12,12,12
hammer curls	3	15,15,15
reverse wrist curls	3	15,15,15

Day 3

exercise	sets	reps
jump squats	3	10,10,10
box steps	3	12,12,12
barbell military press	3	10,10,10
push press	3	12,12,12
squats	3	8,8,8
upright rows	3	12,12,12
front raises	3	15,15,15

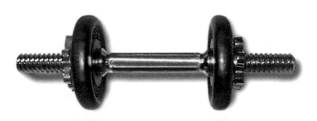

Program Level IV
Endurance/Fat Burning Training
Two-Day Split 4 days per week
Upper & lower body training on the same day
Antagonistic Training

Weeks 1 and 2

Days 1 and 3

exercise	sets	reps
barbell bench press	3	10,10,10
wide-grip pull-ups	2	failure
push press	3	12,12,12
leg curls	3	12,12,12
standing calf raises	3	20,20,20

Days 2 and 4

exercise	sets	reps
leg press	3	12,12,12
power cleans	3	12,12,12
bench dips	2	failure
preacher curls	4	12,12,12,12
reverse curls	3	12,12,12
triceps kickbacks	4	12,12,12

Weeks 3 and 4

Days 1 and 3

exercise	sets	reps
dumbbell bench press	3	12,12,12
close-grip pull-ups	3	failure
push press	3	12,12,12
leg curls	3	15,15,15
standing calf raises	3	20,20,20

Days 2 and 4

exercise	sets	reps
power cleans	3	10,10,10
box steps	3	12,12,12
concentration curls	4	15,15,15,15
triceps curls	4	15,15,15,15
bench dips	3	failure

Program Level IV
Endurance/Fat Burning Training
Two-Day Split 4 days per week
Upper & lower body training on different days

Weeks 1 and 2

Days 1 and 3

exercise	sets	reps
barbell bench press	3	10,10,10
push press	3	12,12,12
wide-grip pull-ups	2	failure
reverse curls	3	15,15,15
dips	2	failure
bent-over dumbbell rows	3	12,12,12

Days 2 and 4

exercise	sets	reps
jump squats	3	10,10,10
power cleans	3	12,12,12
squats	3	8,8,8
lunges	3	10,10,10
box steps	3	12,12,12
standing calf raises	3	20,20,20

Weeks 3 and 4

Days 1 and 3

exercise	sets	reps
dumbbell bench press	3	10,10,10
push press	3	12,12,12
close-grip pull-ups	3	failure
hammer curls	3	15,15,15
cable crossovers	3	10,10,10

Days 2 and 4

exercise	sets	reps
squats	3	8,8,8
lunges	3	10,10,10
jump squats	3	10,10,10
power cleans	3	12,12,12
box steps	3	12,12,12

Program Level IV
Endurance/Fat Burning Training
Two-Day Split 4 days per week
Upper & lower body training on the same day -- Synergistic Training

Weeks 1 and 2

Days 1 and 3

exercise	sets	reps
barbell bench press	3	20
dumbbell incline bench press	2	20
standing flyes	3	20
leg press	3	20
dips	2	failure

Days 2 and 4

exercise	sets	reps
wide-grip pull-ups	2	failure
hammer curls	2	20
leg curls	3	20
standing calf raises	3	20
seated rows	3	20

Weeks 3 and 4

Days 1 and 3

exercise	sets	reps
dumbbell bench press	3	25
incline barbell bench press	2	25
upright rows	3	25
squats	3	25
leg extensions	2	25

Days 2 and 4

exercise	sets	reps
close-grip pull-ups	2	failure
reverse curls	2	25
leg curls	3	25
seated calf raises	2	25
one-arm dumbbell rows	3	25

Program Level V
Endurance/Fat Burning Training
Two-Day Split 4 days per week
Upper & lower body training on the same day -- Antagonistic Training

Weeks 1 and 2

Days 1 and 3

exercise	sets	reps
barbell bench press	3	20
dumbbell military press	3	20
wide-grip pull ups	3	20
leg press	3	20
incline flyes	2	20
lunges	2	20
seated rows	2	20

Days 2 and 4

exercise	sets	reps
leg curls	3	20
standing calf raises	3	20
dumbbell curls	2	20
triceps curls	2	20
hammer curls	2	20
triceps kickbacks	2	20
seated calf raises	2	20

Weeks 3 and 4

Days 1 and 3

exercise	sets	reps
dumbbell bench press	3	25
barbell military press	3	25
close-grip pull downs	3	25
leg curls	2	25
incline barbell bench press	2	25
leg extensions	2	25
dips	3	failure

Days 2 and 4

exercise	sets	reps
squats	3	25
seated calf raises	2	25
barbell curls	2	25
one-arm triceps extension	2	25
reverse curls	2	25
bench dips	3	failure
standing calf raises	3	25

Program Level V
Endurance/Fat Burning Training
Two-Day Split 4 days per week
Upper & lower body training on different days

Weeks 1 and 2

Days 1 and 3

exercise	sets	reps
barbell bench press	3	20,20,20
barbell Military press	3	20,20,20
bent-over dumbbell rows	3	20,20,20
hammer curls	2	20,20
dips	2	failure
wide-grip pull ups	2	failure
cable crossovers	2	20,20

Days 2 and 4

exercise	sets	reps
squats	3	20,20,20
leg press	3	20,20,20
standing calf raises	3	20,20,20
lunges	2	20,20
leg extensions	2	20,20
leg curls	2	20,20
seated calf raises	2	20,20

Weeks 3 and 4

Days 1 and 3

exercise	sets	reps
dumbbell bench press	3	25,25,25
dumbbell military press	3	25,25,25
bent-over barbell rows	3	25,25,25
reverse curls	2	25,25
close-grip pull ups	3	failure
dumbbell curls	2	25,25
incline flyes	2	25,25

Days 2 and 4

exercise	sets	reps
squats	3	25,25,25
leg extensions	2	25,25
leg curls	2	25,25
leg press	3	25,25,25
dead lift	2	25,25
lunges	2	25,25
standing calf raises	3	25,25,25
seated calf raises	2	25,25

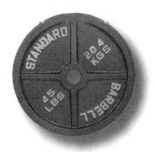

Program Level V
Endurance/Fat Burning Training
Two-Day Split 4 days per week
Upper & lower body training on the same day
Synergistic Training

Weeks 1 and 2

Days 1 and 3

exercise	sets	reps
barbell bench press	3	20
dumbbell incline bench press	2	20
standing flyes	3	20
leg press	3	20
dips	2	failure
lunges	2	20
bench dips	2	failure

Days 2 and 4

exercise	sets	reps
wide-grip pull-ups	2	failure
hammer curls	2	20
leg curls	3	20
standing calf raises	3	20
seated rows	3	20
dumbbell curls	2	20
seated calf raises	2	20

Weeks 3 and 4

Days 1 and 3

exercise	sets	reps
dumbbell bench press	3	25
Incline barbell bench press	2	25
upright rows	3	25
squats	3	25
leg extensions	2	25
bench dips	3	failure
dips	3	failure
front raises	2	25

Days 2 and 4

exercise	sets	reps
close-grip pull-ups	2	failure
reverse curls	2	25
leg curls	3	25
seated calf raises	2	25
one-arm dumbbell rows	3	25
incline dumbbell curls	2	25
standing calf raises	3	25

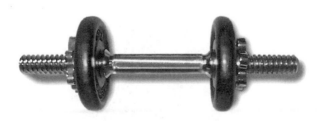

Power/General Fitness Training

Power/General Fitness Training
Entire body every training day
Rest every other day

Weeks 1 and 2

Day 1

exercise	sets	reps
barbell bench press	3	12,12,12
push press	3	10,10,10
wide-grip pull-ups	2	failure
power cleans	3	12,12,12

Day 2

exercise	sets	reps
dumbbell incline bench press	3	12,12,12
upright rows	3	10,10,10
close-grip pull-ups	2	failure

Day 3

exercise	sets	reps
dumbbell bench press	3	12,12,12
push press	3	10,10,10
wide-grip pull-ups	2	failure
power cleans	3	12,12,12

Weeks 3 and 4

Day 1

exercise	sets	reps
barbell bench press	3	12,12,12
push press	3	10,10,10
wide-grip pull-ups	2	failure
power cleans	3	12,12,12

Day 2

exercise	sets	reps
dumbbell incline bench press	3	12,12,12
upright rows	3	10,10,10
close-grip pull-ups	2	failure
leg curls	3	12,12,12

Day 3

exercise	sets	reps
dumbbell bench press	3	12,12,12
push press	3	10,10,10
wide-grip pull-ups	2	failure
power cleans	3	12,12,12

Power/General Fitness Training
Entire body every training day
Rest every other day

Weeks 1 and 2

Day 1

exercise	sets	reps
barbell bench press	3	12,12,12
push press	3	10,10,10
wide-grip pull-ups	2	failure
power cleans	3	12,12,12
jump squats	3	10,10,10

Day 2

exercise	sets	reps
dumbbell incline bench press	3	12,12,12
upright rows	3	10,10,10
close-grip pull-ups	2	failure
leg curls	3	12,12,12
barbell military press	3	10,10,10
standing calf raises	3	20,20,20

Day 3

exercise	sets	reps
dumbbell bench press	3	12,12,12
push press	3	10,10,10
wide-grip pull-ups	2	failure
power cleans	3	12,12,12
box steps	3	10,10,10

Weeks 3 and 4

Day 1

exercise	sets	reps
barbell bench press	3	12,12,12
push press	3	10,10,10
wide-grip pull-ups	2	failure
power cleans	3	12,12,12
jump squats	3	10,10,10

Day 2

exercise	sets	reps
dumbbell incline bench press	3	12,12,12
upright rows	3	10,10,10
close-grip pull-ups	2	failure
leg curls	3	12,12,12
barbell military press	3	10,10,10
standing calf raises	3	20,20,20

Day 3

exercise	sets	reps
dumbbell bench press	3	12,12,12
push press	3	10,10,10
wide-grip pull-ups	2	failure
power cleans	3	12,12,12
box steps	3	10,10,10

Power/General Fitness Training
Three-Day Split four days a week
Antagonistic Training

Weeks 1 and 2

Day 1

exercise	sets	reps
barbell bench press	3	10,10,10
incline dumbbell bench press	3	12,12,12
wide-grip pull-ups	3	failure
T-bar rows	3	10,10,10

Day 2

exercise	sets	reps
bench dips	3	failure
dumbbell triceps curls	3	15,15,15
barbell curls	3	15,15,15
Incline dumbbell curls	3	15,15,15

Day 3

exercise	sets	reps
jump squats	3	10,10,10
power cleans	3	12,12,12
dumbbell military press	3	10,10,10
push press	3	12,12,12

Weeks 3 and 4

Day 1

exercise	sets	reps
dumbbell bench press	3	10,10,10
incline barbell bench press	3	12,12,12
close-grip pull-ups	3	failure
seated cable rows	3	10,10,10

Day 2

exercise	sets	reps
close-grip bench press	3	15,15,15
skull crushers	3	15,15,15
preacher curls	3	15,15,15
concentration curls	3	15,15,15

Day 3

exercise	sets	reps
jump squats	3	10,10,10
box steps	3	12,12,12
barbell military press	3	10,10,10

Power/General Fitness Training
Three-Day Split four days a week
Synergistic Training

Weeks 1 and 2

Day 1

exercise	sets	reps
barbell bench press	3	10,10,10
incline dumbbell bench press	3	12,12,12
bench dips	3	failure
triceps curls	3	15,15,15

Day 2

exercise	sets	reps
wide-grip pull-ups	3	failure
T-bar rows	3	10,10,10
barbell curls	3	15,15,15
incline dumbbell curls	3	15,15,15

Day 3

exercise	sets	reps
jump squats	3	10,10,10
power cleans	3	12,12,12
dumbbell military press	3	10,10,10

Weeks 3 and 4

Day 1

exercise	sets	reps
dumbbell bench press	3	10,10,10
incline barbell bench press	3	12,12,12
close-grip bench press	3	12,12,12
skull crushers	3	15,15,15

Day 2

exercise	sets	reps
close-grip pull-ups	3	failure
seated cable rows	3	10,10,10
preacher curls	3	15,15,15

Day 3

exercise	sets	reps
jump squats	3	10,10,10
box steps	3	12,12,12
barbell military press	3	10,10,10

Program Level III
Power/General Fitness Training
Three-Day Split four days a week
Antagonistic Training

Weeks 1 and 2

Day 1

exercise	sets	reps
barbell bench press	3	10,10,10
dumbbell incline bench press	3	12,12,12
wide-grip pull-ups	3	failure
T-bar rows	3	10,10,10
cable crossovers	3	15,15,15

Day 2

exercise	sets	reps
bench dips	3	failure
barbell triceps curls	3	15,15,15
barbell curls	3	15,15,15
incline dumbbell curls	3	15,15,15
reverse curls	3	15,15,15

Day 3

exercise	sets	reps
jump squats	3	10,10,10
power cleans	3	12,12,12
dumbbell military press	3	10,10,10
push press	3	12,12,12
leg press	3	8,8,8

Weeks 3 and 4

Day 1

exercise	sets	reps
dumbbell bench press	3	10,10,10
incline barbell bench press	3	12,12,12
close-grip pull-ups	3	failure
seated cable rows	3	10,10,10
flyes	3	15,15,15

Day 2

exercise	sets	reps
close-grip bench press	3	15,15,15
skull crushers	3	15,15,15
preacher curls	3	15,15,15
concentration curls	3	15,15,15
hammer curls	3	15,15,15

Day 3

exercise	sets	reps
jump squats	3	10,10,10
box steps	3	12,12,12
barbell military press	3	10,10,10
push press	3	12,12,12
squats	3	8,8,8

Program Level III
Power/General Fitness Training
Three-Day Split four days a week
Synergistic Training

Weeks 1 and 2

Day 1

exercise	sets	reps
barbell bench press	3	10,10,10
incline dumbbell bench press	3	12,12,12
bench dips	3	failure
dumbbell triceps curls	3	15,15,15
cable crossovers	3	15,15,15

Day 2

exercise	sets	reps
wide-grip pull-ups	3	failure
T-bar rows	3	10,10,10
barbell curls	3	15,15,15
incline dumbbell curls	3	15,15,15
one-arm dumbbell rows	3	12,12,12

Day 3

exercise	sets	reps
jump squats	3	10,10,10
power cleans	3	12,12,12
dumbbell military press	3	10,10,10
push press	3	12,12,12
leg press	3	8,8,8

Weeks 3 and 4

Day 1

exercise	sets	reps
dumbbell bench press	3	10,10,10
incline barbell bench press	3	12,12,12
close-grip bench press	3	12,12,12
skull crushers	3	15,15,15
incline flyes	3	15,15,15

Day 2

exercise	sets	reps
close-grip pull-ups	3	failure
seated cable rows	3	10,10,10
preacher curls	3	15,15,15
concentration curls	3	15,15,15
bent-over dumbbell rows	3	12,12,12

Day 3

exercise	sets	reps
jump squats	3	10,10,10
box steps	3	12,12,12
barbell military press	3	10,10,10
push press	3	12,12,12
squats	3	8,8,8

Program Level III
Power/General Fitness Training
Two-Day Split 4 days per week
Upper & lower body training on the same day -- Antagonistic Training

Weeks 1 and 2

Days 1 and 3

exercise	sets	reps
squats	5	10,8,6,4,2
dead lift	5	10,8,6,4,2
preacher curls	4	12,10,8,6
triceps push downs	4	12,10,8,6

Days 2 and 4

exercise	sets	reps
calf raises	3	20,20,20
power cleans	3	12,12,12
bench dips	2	failure
preacher curls	4	12,12,12,12

Weeks 3 and 4

Days 1 and 3

exercise	sets	reps
dumbbell bench press	3	12,12,12
close-grip pull-ups	3	failure
push press	3	12,12,12
leg curls	3	15,15,15

Days 2 and 4

exercise	sets	reps
power cleans	3	10,10,10
box steps	3	12,12,12
concentration curls	4	15,15,15,15
triceps curls	4	15,15,15,15

Program Level III
Power/General Fitness Training
Two-Day Split 4 days per week
Upper & lower body training on different days

Weeks 1 and 2

Days 1 and 3

exercise	sets	reps
barbell bench press	3	10,10,10
push press	3	12,12,12
wide-grip pull-ups	2	failure
reverse curls	3	15,15,15

Days 2 and 4

exercise	sets	reps
jump squats	3	10,10,10
cleans	3	12,12,12
lunges	3	10,10,10
standing calf raises	3	20,20,20

Weeks 3 and 4

Days 1 and 3

exercise	sets	reps
dumbbell bench press	3	10,10,10
push press	3	12,12,12
close-grip pull-ups	3	failure
hammer curls	3	15,15,15

Days 2 and 4

exercise	sets	reps
lunges	3	10,10,10
jump squats	3	10,10,10
power cleans	3	12,12,12
standing calf raises	3	20,20,20

Power/General Fitness Training
Two-Day Split 4 days per week
Upper & lower body training on the same day -- Synergistic Training

Weeks 1 and 2

Days 1 and 3

exercise	sets	reps
dumbbell bench press	3	10,10,10
push press	3	12,12,12
dumbbell incline bench press	3	12,12,12
leg curls	3	12,12,12

Days 2 and 4

exercise	sets	reps
wide-grip pull-ups	2	failure
reverse curls	3	12,12,12
squats	4	10,10,10
box steps	3	12,12,12

Weeks 3 and 4

Days 1 and 3

exercise	sets	reps
barbell bench press	3	12,12,12
push press	3	12,12,12
incline barbell bench press	3	12,12,12
standing calf raises	3	20,20,20

Days 2 and 4

exercise	sets	reps
close-grip pull-ups	3	failure
hammer curls	4	12,12,12,12
jump squats	3	10,10,10
power cleans	3	12,12,12

Program Level III
Power/General Fitness Training
Entire body every training day -- Rest every other day

Weeks 1 and 2

Day 1

exercise	sets	reps
barbell bench press	3	12,12,12
push press	3	10,10,10
wide-grip pull-ups	2	failure
power cleans	3	12,12,12
jump squats	3	10,10,10
standing flyes	3	15,15,15
T-bar rows	3	12,12,12

Day 2

exercise	sets	reps
dumbbell incline bench press	3	12,12,12
upright rows	3	10,10,10
close-grip pull-ups	2	failure
leg curls	3	12,12,12
barbell military press	3	10,10,10
standing calf raises	3	20,20,20
seated cable rows	3	12,12,12

Day 3

exercise	sets	reps
dumbbell bench press	3	12,12,12
push press	3	10,10,10
wide-grip pull-ups	2	failure
power cleans	3	12,12,12
box steps	3	10,10,10
standing flyes	3	15,15,15
T-bar rows	3	12,12,12

Weeks 3 and 4

Day 1

exercise	sets	reps
barbell bench press	3	12,12,12
push press	3	10,10,10
wide-grip pull-ups	2	failure
power cleans	3	12,12,12
jump squats	3	10,10,10
standing flyes	3	15,15,15
T-bar rows	3	12,12,12

Day 2

exercise	sets	reps
dumbbell incline bench press	3	12,12,12
upright rows	3	10,10,10
close-grip pull-ups	2	failure
leg curls	3	12,12,12
barbell military press	3	10,10,10
standing calf raises	3	20,20,20
seated cable rows	3	12,12,12

Day 3

exercise	sets	reps
dumbbell bench press	3	12,12,12
push press	3	10,10,10
wide-grip pull-ups	2	failure
power cleans	3	12,12,12
box steps	3	10,10,10
standing flyes	3	15,15,15
T-bar rows	3	12,12,12

Program Level IV
Power/General Fitness Training
Three-Day Split four days a week -- Antagonistic Training

Weeks 1 and 2

Day 1

exercise	sets	reps
barbell bench press	3	10,10,10
incline dumbbell bench press	3	12,12,12
wide-grip pull-ups	3	failure
T-bar rows	3	10,10,10
cable crossovers	3	15,15,15
one-arm dumbbell rows	3	12,12,12
dips	3	failure

Day 2

exercise	sets	reps
bench dips	3	failure
dumbbell triceps curls	3	15,15,15
barbell curls	3	15,15,15
incline dumbbell curls	3	15,15,15
reverse curls	3	15,15,15
one-arm triceps extensions	3	15,15,15
behind back wrist curls	3	15,15,15

Day 3

exercise	sets	reps
jump squats	3	10,10,10
power cleans	3	12,12,12
dumbbell military press	3	10,10,10
push press	3	12,12,12
leg press	3	8,8,8
bent-over lateral raises	3	15,15,15
standing flyes	3	12,12,12

Weeks 3 and 4

Day 1

exercise	sets	reps
jump squats	3	10,10,10
power cleans	3	12,12,12
dumbbell military press	3	10,10,10
push press	3	12,12,12
leg press	3	8,8,8
bent-over lateral raises	3	15,15,15
standing flyes	3	12,12,12

Day 2

exercise	sets	reps
close-grip bench press	3	15,15,15
skull crushers	3	15,15,15
preacher curls	3	15,15,15
concentration curls	3	15,15,15
hammer curls	3	15,15,15
triceps push downs	3	15,15,15
reverse wrist curls	3	15,15,15

Day 3

exercise	sets	reps
jump squats	3	10,10,10
box steps	3	12,12,12
barbell military press	3	10,10,10
push press	3	12,12,12
squats	3	8,8,8
upright rows	3	12,12,12
front raises	3	15,15,15

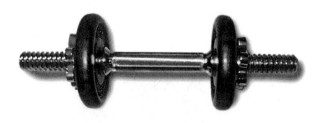

Program Level IV
Power/General Fitness Training
Three-Day Split four days a week -- Synergistic Training

Weeks 1 and 2

Day 1

exercise	sets	reps
barbell bench press	3	10,10,10
dumbbell incline bench press	3	12,12,12
bench dips	3	failure
dumbbells triceps curls	3	15,15,15
cable crossovers	3	15,15,15
one-arm triceps extensions	3	15,15,15
dips	3	failure

Day 2

exercise	sets	reps
wide-grip lat pull down	3	10,10,10
T-bar row	3	12,12,12
barbell curls	3	failure
concentration curls	3	15,15,15
seated cable rows	3	15,15,15
bent-over barbell rows	3	15,15,15
hammer curls	3	12,12,12

Day 3

exercise	sets	reps
jump squats	3	10,10,10
power cleans	3	12,12,12
dumbbell military press	3	10,10,10
push press	3	12,12,12
leg press	3	8,8,8
bent-over lateral raises	3	15,15,15
standing flyes	3	12,12,12

Weeks 3 and 4

Day 1

exercise	sets	reps
dumbbell bench press	3	10,10,10
incline barbell bench press	3	12,12,12
close-grip bench press	3	12,12,12
skull crushers	3	15,15,15
incline flyes	3	15,15,15
triceps push downs	3	15,15,15
dips	3	failure

Day 2

exercise	sets	reps
close-grip pull-ups	3	failure
seated cable rows	3	10,10,10
preacher curls	3	15,15,15
concentration curls	3	15,15,15
bent-over dumbbell rows	3	12,12,12
hammer curls	3	15,15,15
reverse wrist curls	3	15,15,15
close-grip lat pull downs	3	12,12,12

Day 3

exercise	sets	reps
jump squats	3	10,10,10
box steps	3	12,12,12
barbell military press	3	10,10,10
push press	3	12,12,12
squats	3	8,8,8
upright rows	3	12,12,12
front raises	3	15,15,15

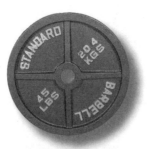

Program Level IV
Power/General Fitness Training
Two-Day Split 4 days per week
Upper & lower body training on the same day -- Antagonistic Training

Weeks 1 and 2

Days 1 and 3

exercise	sets	reps
barbell bench press	3	10,10,10
wide-grip pull-ups	2	failure
push press	3	12,12,12
leg curls	3	12,12,12
standing calf raises	3	20,20,20

Days 2 and 4

exercise	sets	reps
leg press	3	12,12,12
power cleans	3	12,12,12
bench dips	2	failure
preacher curls	4	12,12,12,12
reverse curls	3	12,12,12

Weeks 3 and 4

Days 1 and 3

exercise	sets	reps
dumbbell bench press	3	12,12,12
close-grip pull-ups	3	failure
push press	3	12,12,12
leg curls	3	15,15,15
standing calf raises	3	20,20,20

Days 2 and 4

exercise	sets	reps
power cleans	3	10,10,10
box steps	3	12,12,12
concentration curls	4	15,15,15,15
triceps curls	4	15,15,15,15
bench dips	3	failure

Program Level IV
Power/General Fitness Training
Two-Day Split 4 days per week
Upper & lower body training on different days

Weeks 1 and 2

Days 1 and 3

exercise	sets	reps
barbell bench press	3	10,10,10
push press	3	12,12,12
wide-grip pull-ups	2	failure
reverse curls	3	15,15,15
dips	2	failure

Days 2 and 4

exercise	sets	reps
jump squats	3	10,10,10
power cleans	3	12,12,12
squats	3	8,8,8
lunges	3	10,10,10
box steps	3	12,12,12

Weeks 3 and 4

Days 1 and 3

exercise	sets	reps
dumbbell bench press	3	10,10,10
push press	3	12,12,12
close-grip pull-ups	3	failure
hammer curls	3	15,15,15
cable crossovers	3	10,10,10
T-bar rows	3	12,12,12

Days 2 and 4

exercise	sets	reps
squats	3	8,8,8
lunges	3	10,10,10
jump squats	3	10,10,10
power cleans	3	12,12,12
box steps	3	12,12,12

Program Level IV
Power/General Fitness Training
Two-Day Split 4 days per week
Upper & lower body training on the same day -- Synergistic Training

Weeks 1 and 2

Days 1 and 3

exercise	sets	reps
dumbbell bench press	3	10,10,10
push press	3	12,12,12
dumbbell incline bench press	3	12,12,12
leg curls	3	12,12,12
dips	2	failure

Days 2 and 4

exercise	sets	reps
wide-grip pull-ups	2	failure
reverse curls	3	12,12,12
squats	4	10,10,10
box steps	3	12,12,12
T-bar rows	3	12,12,12

Weeks 3 and 4

Days 1 and 3

exercise	sets	reps
barbell bench press	3	12,12,12
push press	3	12,12,12
incline barbell bench press	3	12,12,12
standing calf raises	3	20,20,20
leg curls	4	10,10,10
bench dips	3	failure

Days 2 and 4

exercise	sets	reps
close-grip pull-ups	3	failure
hammer curls	4	12,12,12,12
jump squats	3	10,10,10
power cleans	3	12,12,12
box steps	3	12,12,12

Program Level V
Power/General Fitness Training
Two-Day Split 4 days per week
Upper & lower body training on the same day -- Antagonistic Training

Weeks 1 and 2

Days 1 and 3

exercise	sets	reps
barbell bench press	3	10,10,10
wide-grip pull-ups	2	failure
push press	3	12,12,12
leg curls	3	12,12,12
standing calf raises	3	20,20,20
dips	2	failure
one-arm dumbbell rows	3	12,12,12

Days 2 and 4

exercise	sets	reps
leg press	3	12,12,12
power cleans	3	12,12,12
bench dips	2	failure
preacher curls	4	12,12,12,12
reverse curls	3	12,12,12
triceps kickbacks	4	12,12,12
leg extension	3	15,15,15

Weeks 3 and 4

Days 1 and 3

exercise	sets	reps
dumbbell bench press	3	12,12,12
close-grip pull-ups	3	failure
push press	3	12,12,12
leg curls	3	15,15,15
standing calf raises	3	20,20,20
dips	3	failure
cable crossovers	3	10,10,10

Days 2 and 4

exercise	sets	reps
power cleans	3	10,10,10
box steps	3	12,12,12
concentration curls	4	15,15,15,15
triceps curls	4	15,15,15,15
bench dips	3	failure
hammer curls	3	12,12,12
jump squats	3	12,12,12

Program Level V
Power/General Fitness Training
Two-Day Split 4 days per week
Upper & lower body training on different days

Weeks 1 and 2

Days 1 and 3

exercise	sets	reps
barbell bench press	3	10,10,10
push press	3	12,12,12
wide-grip pull-ups	2	failure
reverse curls	3	15,15,15
dips	2	failure
bent-over dumbbell rows	3	12,12,12
incline flyes	3	12,12,12

Days 2 and 4

exercise	sets	reps
jump squats	3	10,10,10
power cleans	3	12,12,12
squats	3	8,8,8
lunges	3	10,10,10
box steps	3	12,12,12
leg curls	3	12,12,12
leg extensions	3	12,12,12

Weeks 3 and 4

Days 1 and 3

exercise	sets	reps
dumbbell bench press	3	10,10,10
push press	3	12,12,12
close-grip pull-ups	3	failure
hammer curls	3	15,15,15
cable crossovers	3	10,10,10
T-bar rows	3	12,12,12
incline bench press	3	12,12,12

Days 2 and 4

exercise	sets	reps
squats	3	8,8,8
box steps	3	12,12,12
power cleans	3	12,12,12
jump squats	3	10,10,10
lunges	3	10,10,10
leg curls	3	12,12,12
leg extensions	3	12,12,12

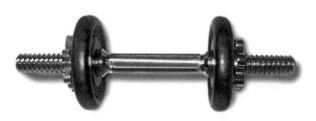

Program Level V
Power/General Fitness Training
Two-Day Split 4 days per week
Upper & lower body training on the same day

Weeks 1 and 2

Days 1 and 3

exercise	sets	reps
dumbbell bench press	3	10,10,10
push press	3	12,12,12
dumbbell incline bench press	3	12,12,12
leg curls	3	12,12,12
dips	2	failure
standing calf raises	3	20,20,20
bench dips	2	failure

Days 2 and 4

exercise	sets	reps
dumbbell bench press	3	10,10,10
push press	3	12,12,12
dumbbell incline bench press	3	12,12,12
leg curls	3	12,12,12
dips	2	failure
standing calf raises	3	20,20,20
behind the neck pull downs	3	12,12,12

Weeks 3 and 4

Days 1 and 3

exercise	sets	reps
barbell bench press	3	12,12,12
push press	3	12,12,12
incline barbell bench press	3	12,12,12
standing calf raises	3	20,20,20
leg curls	4	10,10,10
bench dips	3	failure
dips	3	failure

Days 2 and 4

exercise	sets	reps
close-grip pull-ups	3	failure
hammer curls	4	12,12,12,12
jump squats	3	10,10,10
power cleans	3	12,12,12
box steps	3	12,12,12
one-arm dumbbell rows	3	12,12,12
T-bar rows	3	10,10,10

Strength Training

Program Level I

Strength Training

Entire body every training day
Rest every other day

Weeks 1 and 2

Day 1

exercise	sets	reps
barbell bench press	5	8,6,4,2,1
barbell military press	5	8,6,4,2,1
wide-grip lat pull downs	4	8,8,8,8

Day 2

exercise	sets	reps
incline barbell bench press	5	8,6,4,2,1
barbell military press	5	8,6,4,2,1
close-grip lat pull downs	4	8,8,8,8
leg press	5	10,8,6,4,2

Day 3

exercise	sets	reps
barbell bench press	5	8,6,4,2,1
barbell military press	5	8,6,4,2,1
wide-grip lat pull downs	4	8,8,8,8
squats	5	10,8,6,4,2

Weeks 3 and 4

Day 1

exercise	sets	reps
barbell bench press	5	8,6,4,2,1
barbell military press	5	8,6,4,2,1
T-bar rows	4	8,8,8,8
leg press	5	10,8,6,4,2

Day 2

exercise	sets	reps
incline barbell bench press	5	8,6,4,2,1
barbell military press	5	8,6,4,2,1
seated cable rows	4	8,8,8,8
squats	5	10,8,6,4,2

Day 3

exercise	sets	reps
barbell bench press	5	8,6,4,2,1
barbell military press	5	8,6,4,2,1
bent-over barbell rows	4	8,8,8,8
leg press	5	10,8,6,4,2

Program Level II

Strength Training

Three-Day Split four days a week
Antagonistic Training

Weeks 1 and 2

Day 1

exercise	sets	reps
barbell bench press	5	8,6,4,2,1
incline barbell bench press	5	8,6,4,2,1
wide-grip lat pull downs	4	8,8,8,8
seated cable rows	4	8,8,8,8

Day 2

exercise	sets	reps
squats	5	10,8,6,4,2
leg press	5	10,8,6,4,2
barbell military press	5	8,6,4,2,1
upright rows	4	8,8,6,6

Day 3

exercise	sets	reps
barbell triceps curls	5	12,10,8,6,2
close-grip barbell bench press	5	12,10,8,6,2
hammer curls	4	12,10,8,6
preacher curls	4	12,10,8,6

Weeks 3 and 4

Day 1

exercise	sets	reps
barbell bench press	5	8,6,4,2,1
incline barbell bench press	5	8,6,4,2,1
close-grip lat pull downs	4	8,8,8,8
T-bar rows	4	8,8,8,8

Day 2

exercise	sets	reps
squats	5	10,8,6,4,2
dead lift	5	10,8,6,4,2
barbell military press	5	8,6,4,2,1
standing flyes	4	8,8,6,6

Day 3

exercise	sets	reps
barbell triceps curls	5	12,10,8,6,2
triceps push downs	5	12,10,8,6,2
reverse barbell curls	4	12,10,8,6
barbell curls	4	12,10,8,6

Strength Training
Three-Day Split four days a week
Synergistic Training

Weeks 1 and 2

Day 1

exercise	sets	reps
barbell bench press	5	8,6,4,2,1
incline barbell bench press	5	8,6,4,2,1
close-grip barbell bench press	5	8,6,4,2,1
triceps push downs	4	12,10,8,6

Day 2

exercise	sets	reps
wide-grip lat pull downs	4	8,8,8,8
hammer curls	4	12,10,8,6
preacher curls	4	12,10,8,6

Day 3

exercise	sets	reps
squats	5	10,8,6,4,2
leg press	5	10,8,6,4,2
barbell military press	5	8,6,4,2,1

Weeks 3 and 4

Day 1

exercise	sets	reps
incline barbell bench press	5	8,6,4,2,1
barbell triceps curls	4	12,10,8,6
flyes	4	8,8,6,6

Day 2

exercise	sets	reps
close-grip lat pull downs	4	8,8,8,8
reverse barbell curls	4	12,10,8,6
T-bar rows	4	8,8,8,8

Day 3

exercise	sets	reps
squats	5	10,8,6,4,2
barbell military press	5	8,6,4,2,1
standing flyes	4	8,8,6,6
dead lift	5	10,8,6,4,2

Strength Training
Entire body every training day
Rest every other day

Weeks 1 and 2

Day 1

exercise	sets	reps
barbell bench press	5	8,6,4,2,1
barbell military press	5	8,6,4,2,1
wide-grip lat pull downs	4	8,8,8,8
squats	5	10,8,6,4,2
incline barbell bench press	4	8,6,4,2

Day 2

exercise	sets	reps
incline barbell bench press	5	8,6,4,2,1
barbell military press	5	8,6,4,2,1
close-grip lat pull downs	4	8,8,8,8
leg press	5	10,8,6,4,2
barbell bench press	4	8,6,4,2

Day 3

exercise	sets	reps
barbell bench press	5	8,6,4,2,1
barbell military press	5	8,6,4,2,1
wide-grip lat pull downs	4	8,8,8,8
squats	5	10,8,6,4,2
incline dumbbell bench press	4	8,6,4,2

Weeks 3 and 4

Day 1

exercise	sets	reps
barbell bench press	5	8,6,4,2,1
barbell military press	5	8,6,4,2,1
T-bar rows	4	8,8,8,8
leg press	5	10,8,6,4,2
incline barbell bench press	4	8,6,4,2
dead lift	5	10,8,6,4,2

Day 2

exercise	sets	reps
incline barbell bench press	5	8,6,4,2,1
barbell military press	5	8,6,4,2,1
seated cable rows	4	8,8,8,8
squats	5	10,8,6,4,2
incline flyes	4	8,6,4,2

Day 3

exercise	sets	reps
barbell bench press	5	8,6,4,2,1
barbell military press	5	8,6,4,2,1
bent-over barbell rows	4	8,8,8,8
leg press	5	10,8,6,4,2
incline barbell bench press	4	8,6,4,2

Program Level III

Strength Training

Three-Day Split four days a week -- Antagonistic Training

Weeks 1 and 2

Day 1

exercise	sets	reps
barbell bench press	5	8,6,4,2,1
incline barbell bench press	5	8,6,4,2,1
wide-grip lat pull downs	4	8,8,8,8
seated cable rows	4	8,8,8,8
cable crossovers	4	8,8,6,6
bent-over barbell rows	4	8,8,8,8

Day 2

exercise	sets	reps
squats	5	10,8,6,4,2
leg press	5	10,8,6,4,2
barbell military press	5	8,6,4,2,1
upright rows	4	8,8,6,6
lunges	4	10,8,8,6

Day 3

exercise	sets	reps
barbell triceps curls	5	12,10,8,6,2
close-grip barbell bench press	5	12,10,8,6,2
hammer curls	4	12,10,8,6
preacher curls	4	12,10,8,6
bench dips	5	12,10,8,6,2

Weeks 3 and 4

Day 1

exercise	sets	reps
barbell bench press	5	8,6,4,2,1
incline barbell bench press	5	8,6,4,2,1
close-grip lat pull downs	4	8,8,8,8
T-bar rows	4	8,8,8,8
flyes	4	10,8,8,6

Day 2

exercise	sets	reps
squats	5	10,8,6,4,2
dead lift	5	10,8,6,4,2
barbell military press	5	8,6,4,2,1
standing flyes	4	8,8,6,6
lunges	4	10,8,8,6

Day 3

exercise	sets	reps
barbell triceps curls	5	12,10,8,6,2
triceps push downs	5	12,10,8,6,2
reverse barbell curls	4	12,10,8,6
barbell curls	4	12,10,8,6
dips	5	12,10,8,6,2

Program Level III

Strength Training

Three-Day Split four days a week -- Synergistic Training

Weeks 1 and 2

Day 1

exercise	sets	reps
barbell bench press	5	8,6,4,2,1
incline barbell bench press	5	8,6,4,2,1
close-grip barbell bench press	5	8,6,4,2,1
triceps push downs	4	12,10,8,6
flyes	4	10,8,8,6

Day 2

exercise	sets	reps
wide-grip lat pull downs	4	8,8,8,8
hammer curls	4	12,10,8,6
preacher curls	4	12,10,8,6
bent-over barbell rows	4	8,8,8,8
seated cable rows	4	8,8,8,8

Day 3

exercise	sets	reps
squats	5	10,8,6,4,2
leg press	5	10,8,6,4,2
barbell military press	5	8,6,4,2,1
upright rows	4	8,8,6,6
lunges	4	10,8,8,6

Weeks 3 and 4

Day 1

exercise	sets	reps
barbell bench press	5	8,6,4,2,1
incline barbell bench press	5	8,6,4,2,1
triceps kickbacks	5	8,6,4,2,1
triceps pull downs	4	12,10,8,6
incline flyes	4	10,8,8,6

Day 2

exercise	sets	reps
close-grip lat pull downs	4	8,8,8,8
reverse barbell curls	4	12,10,8,6
incline dumbbell curls	4	12,10,8,6
behind the neck pull downs	4	8,8,8,8
T-bar rows	4	8,8,8,8

Day 3

exercise	sets	reps
squats	5	10,8,6,4,2
dead lift	5	10,8,6,4,2
barbell military press	5	8,6,4,2,1
lateral raises	4	8,8,8,8
leg curls	4	10,8,8,6

Program Level III
Strength Training
Two-Day Split 4 days per week
Upper & lower body training on the same day -- Antagonistic Training

Weeks 1 and 2

Days 1 and 3

exercise	sets	reps
barbell bench press	5	8,6,4,2,1
wide-grip lat pull downs	4	8,8,8,8
barbell military press	5	8,6,4,2,1
leg curls	5	10,8,6,4,2

Days 2 and 4

exercise	sets	reps
squats	5	10,8,6,4,2
leg press	5	10,8,6,4,2
barbell curls	4	12,10,8,6
skull crushers	5	12,10,8,6,2

Weeks 3 and 4

Days 1 and 3

exercise	sets	reps
barbell bench press	5	8,6,4,2,1
close-grip lat pull downs	4	8,8,8,8
barbell military press	5	8,6,4,2,1
leg curls	5	10,8,6,4,2

Days 2 and 4

exercise	sets	reps
squats	5	10,8,6,4,2
dead lift	5	10,8,6,4,2
preacher curls	4	12,10,8,6
triceps push downs	4	12,10,8,6

Program Level III
Strength Training
Two-Day Split 4 days per week
Upper & lower body training on different days

Weeks 1 and 2

Days 1 and 3

exercise	sets	reps
barbell bench press	5	8,6,4,2,1
wide-grip lat pull downs	4	8,8,8,8
barbell military press	5	8,6,4,2,1
hammer curls	4	12,10,8,6

Days 2 and 4

exercise	sets	reps
squats	5	10,8,6,4,2
leg press	5	10,8,6,4,2
lunges	5	10,8,6,4,2

Weeks 3 and 4

Days 1 and 3

exercise	sets	reps
barbell bench press	5	8,6,4,2,1
close-grip lat pull downs	4	8,8,8,8
barbell military press	5	8,6,4,2,1
reverse curls	4	12,10,8,6

Days 2 and 4

exercise	sets	reps
leg press	5	10,8,6,4,2
Leg extensions	5	10,8,6,4,2
squats	5	10,8,6,4,2
seated calf raises	4	20,20,20,20

Program Level III
Strength Training
Two-Day Split 4 days per week
Upper & lower body training on the same day -- Synergistic Training

Weeks 1 and 2

Days 1 and 3

exercise	sets	reps
barbell bench press	5	8,6,4,2,1
upright rows	5	8,6,4,2,1
incline barbell bench press	5	8,6,4,2,1
leg curls	5	10,8,6,4,2

Days 2 and 4

exercise	sets	reps
wide-grip lat pull downs	4	8,8,8,8
hammer curls	4	12,10,8,6
squats	5	10,8,6,4,2
leg extensions	4	8,8,6,6

Weeks 3 and 4

Days 1 and 3

exercise	sets	reps
barbell bench press	5	8,6,4,2,1
upright rows	5	8,6,4,2,1
incline barbell bench press	5	8,6,4,2,1
leg curls	5	10,8,6,4,2

Days 2 and 4

exercise	sets	reps
close-grip lat pull downs	4	8,8,8,8
reverse curls	4	12,10,8,6
leg press	5	10,8,6,4,2

Program Level III
Strength Training
Entire body every training day -- Rest every other day

Weeks 1 and 2

Day 1

exercise	sets	reps
barbell bench press	5	8,6,4,2,1
barbell military press	5	8,6,4,2,1
wide-grip lat pull downs	4	8,8,8,8
squats	5	10,8,6,4,2
incline barbell bench press	4	8,6,4,2
lunges	4	10,8,8,6
bent-over barbell rows	4	8,8,8,8

Day 2

exercise	sets	reps
incline barbell bench press	5	8,6,4,2,1
barbell military press	5	8,6,4,2,1
close-grip lat pull downs	4	8,8,8,8
leg press	5	10,8,6,4,2
barbell bench press	4	8,6,4,2
dead lift	5	10,8,6,4,2
seated cable rows	4	8,8,8,8

Day 3

exercise	sets	reps
barbell bench press	5	8,6,4,2,1
barbell military press	5	8,6,4,2,1
wide-grip lat pull downs	4	8,8,8,8
squats	5	10,8,6,4,2
incline barbell bench press	4	8,6,4,2
lunges	4	10,8,8,6
bent-over barbell rows	4	8,8,8,8

Weeks 3 and 4

Day 1

exercise	sets	reps
barbell bench press	5	8,6,4,2,1
barbell military press	5	8,6,4,2,1
T-bar rows	4	8,8,8,8
leg press	5	10,8,6,4,2
incline barbell bench press	4	8,6,4,2
dead lift	5	10,8,6,4,2
wide-grip lat pull downs	4	8,8,8,8

Day 2

exercise	sets	reps
incline barbell bench press	5	8,6,4,2,1
barbell military press	5	8,6,4,2,1
seated cable rows	4	8,8,8,8
squats	5	10,8,6,4,2
incline flyes	4	8,6,4,2
lunges	5	10,8,6,4,2
close-grip lat pull downs	4	8,8,8,8

Day 3

exercise	sets	reps
barbell bench press	5	8,6,4,2,1
barbell military press	5	8,6,4,2,1
bent-over barbell rows	4	8,8,8,8
leg press	5	10,8,6,4,2
incline barbell bench press	4	8,6,4,2
dead lift	5	10,8,6,4,2
wide-grip lat pull downs	4	8,8,8,8

Program Level IV
Strength Training
Two-Day Split 4 days per week
Upper & lower body training on different days

Weeks 1 and 2

Days 1 and 3

exercise	sets	reps
barbell bench press	5	8,6,4,2,1
wide-grip lat pull downs	4	8,8,8,8
barbell military press	5	8,6,4,2,1
hammer curls	4	12,10,8,6
close-grip barbell bench press	4	10,10,8,8

Days 2 and 4

exercise	sets	reps
squats	5	10,8,6,4,2
leg press	5	10,8,6,4,2
leg curls	4	8,8,6,6
lunges	4	10,8,8,6
leg extensions	4	8,8,6,6

Weeks 3 and 4

Days 1 and 3

exercise	sets	reps
barbell bench press	5	8,6,4,2,1
close-grip lat pull downs	4	8,8,8,8
barbell military press	5	8,6,4,2,1
reverse curls	4	12,10,8,6
incline barbell bench press	4	10,10,8,8

Days 2 and 4

exercise	sets	reps
leg press	5	10,8,6,4,2
squats	5	10,8,6,4,2
lunges	4	10,8,6,4,2
leg extensions	4	10,8,8,6
leg curls	4	8,8,6,6

Program Level IV
Strength Training
Three-Day Split four days a week -- Antagonistic Training

Weeks 1 and 2

Day 1

exercise	sets	reps
barbell bench press	5	8,6,4,2,1
incline barbell bench press	5	8,6,4,2,1
wide-grip lat pull downs	4	8,8,8,8
seated cable rows	4	8,8,8,8
cable crossovers	4	8,8,6,6
bent-over barbell rows	4	8,8,8,8
incline flyes	4	10,8,6,6

Day 2

exercise	sets	reps
squats	5	10,8,6,4,2
leg press	5	10,8,6,4,2
barbell military press	5	8,6,4,2,1
upright rows	4	8,8,6,6
lunges	4	10,8,8,6
barbell shrugs	4	10,8,8,6
dead lift	5	10,8,6,4,2

Day 3

exercise	sets	reps
barbell triceps curls	5	12,10,8,6,2
close-grip barbell bench press	5	12,10,8,6,2
hammer curls	4	12,10,8,6
preacher curls	4	12,10,8,6
bench dips	5	12,10,8,6,2
barbell curls	4	12,10,8,6
skull crushers	5	12,10,8,6,2

Weeks 3 and 4

Day 1

exercise	sets	reps
barbell bench press	5	8,6,4,2,1
incline barbell bench press	5	8,6,4,2,1
close-grip lat pull downs	4	8,8,8,8
T-bar rows	4	8,8,8,8
flyes	4	10,8,8,6
behind the neck pull downs	4	8,8,8,8
cable crossovers	4	10,8,8,6

Day 2

exercise	sets	reps
squats	5	10,8,6,4,2
dead lift	5	10,8,6,4,2
barbell military press	5	8,6,4,2,1
standing flyes	4	8,8,6,6
lunges	4	10,8,8,6
barbell shrugs	4	10,8,8,6
leg press	5	10,8,6,4,2

Day 3

exercise	sets	reps
barbell triceps curls	5	12,10,8,6,2
triceps push downs	5	12,10,8,6,2
reverse barbell curls	4	12,10,8,6
barbell curls	4	12,10,8,6
dips	5	12,10,8,6,2
preacher curls	4	12,10,8,6
skull crushers	5	12,10,8,6,2

Program Level IV
Strength Training
Three-Day Split four days a week -- Synergistic Training
Weeks 1 and 2

Day 1

exercise	sets	reps
barbell bench press	5	8,6,4,2,1
incline barbell bench press	5	8,6,4,2,1
close-grip barbell bench press	5	8,6,4,2,1
triceps push downs	4	12,10,8,6
flyes	4	10,8,8,6
skull crushers	5	12,10,8,6,2
dips	4	8,8,8,8

Day 2

exercise	sets	reps
wide-grip lat pull downs	4	8,8,8,8
hammer curls	4	12,10,8,6
preacher curls	4	12,10,8,6
bent-over barbell rows	4	8,8,8,8
seated cable rows	4	8,8,8,8
barbell curls	4	12,10,8,6
incline dumbbell curls	4	12,10,8,6

Day 3

exercise	sets	reps
squats	5	10,8,6,4,2
leg press	5	10,8,6,4,2
barbell military press	5	8,6,4,2,1
upright rows	4	8,8,6,6
lunges	4	10,8,8,6
standing flyes	4	8,8,6,6
leg extensions	4	8,8,6,6

Weeks 3 and 4

Day 1

exercise	sets	reps
barbell bench press	5	8,6,4,2,1
incline barbell bench press	5	8,6,4,2,1
dumbbell triceps curls	4	8,6,6,6
triceps pull downs	4	12,10,8,6
incline flyes	4	10,8,8,6
one-arm triceps extensions	5	12,10,8,6,2
bench dips	4	8,8,8,8

Day 2

exercise	sets	reps
close-grip lat pull downs	4	8,8,8,8
reverse barbell curls	4	12,10,8,6
concentration curls	4	12,10,8,6
behind the neck pull downs	4	8,8,8,8
seated cable rows	4	8,8,8,8
barbell curls	4	12,10,8,6
dumbbell curls	4	12,10,8,6

Day 3

exercise	sets	reps
squats	5	10,8,6,4,2
dead lift	5	10,8,6,4,2
barbell military press	5	8,6,4,2,1
upright rows	4	8,8,6,6
leg curls	4	10,8,8,6
standing flyes	4	8,8,6,6
standing calf raises	4	20,20,20,20

Program Level IV
Strength Training
Two-Day Split 4 days per week -- Upper & lower body training on the same day -- Antagonistic Training
Weeks 1 and 2

Days 1 and 3

exercise	sets	reps
barbell bench press	5	8,6,4,2,1
wide-grip lat pull downs	4	8,8,8,8
incline barbell bench press	5	8,6,4,2,1
barbell military press	5	10,8,6,4,2
leg curls	5	8,6,4,2,1

Days 2 and 4

exercise	sets	reps
squats	5	10,8,6,4,2
leg press	5	10,8,6,4,2
barbell curls	4	12,10,8,6
skull crushers	5	12,10,8,6,2
hammer curls	4	12,10,8,6

Weeks 3 and 4

Days 1 and 3

exercise	sets	reps
barbell bench press	5	8,6,4,2,1
close-grip lat pull downs	4	8,8,8,8
barbell military press	5	8,6,4,2,1
leg curls	5	10,8,6,4,2
good mornings	4	15,15,15,15

Days 2 and 4

exercise	sets	reps
squats	5	10,8,6,4,2
dead lift	5	10,8,6,4,2
preacher curls	4	12,10,8,6
triceps push downs	4	12,10,8,6
reverse curls	4	12,10,8,6

Program Level IV
Strength Training
Two-Day Split 4 days per week

Upper & lower body training on the same day
Synergistic Training

Weeks 1 and 2

Days 1 and 3

exercise	sets	reps
barbell bench press	5	8,6,4,2,1
barbell military press	5	8,6,4,2,1
incline barbell bench press	5	8,6,4,2,1
leg curls	5	10,8,6,4,2
close grip barbell bench press	4	10,10,8,8

Days 2 and 4

exercise	sets	reps
wide-grip lat pull downs	4	8,8,8,8
hammer curls	4	12,10,8,6
squats	5	10,8,6,4,2
leg extensions	4	8,8,6,6
bent-over rows	4	8,8,8,8

Weeks 3 and 4

Days 1 and 3

exercise	sets	reps
barbell bench press	5	8,6,4,2,1
barbell military press	5	8,6,4,2,1
incline barbell bench press	5	8,6,4,2,1
leg curls	5	10,8,6,4,2
barbell triceps curls	4	10,10,8,8

Days 2 and 4

exercise	sets	reps
close-grip lat pull downs	4	8,8,8,8
reverse curls	4	12,10,8,6
leg press	5	10,8,6,4,2
leg extensions	4	8,8,6,6
bent-over barbell rows	4	8,8,8,8

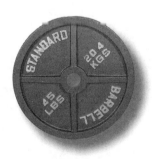

Program Level V
Strength Training
Two-Day Split 4 days per week

Upper & lower body training on the same day
Antagonistic Training

Weeks 1 and 2

Days 1 and 3

exercise	sets	reps
barbell bench press	5	8,6,4,2,1
wide-grip lat pull downs	4	8,8,8,8
barbell military press	5	8,6,4,2,1
leg curls	5	10,8,6,4,2
incline barbell bench press	5	8,6,4,2,1
standing calf raises	4	20,20,20,20
T-bar rows	4	8,8,8,8

Days 2 and 4

exercise	sets	reps
squats	5	10,8,6,4,2
leg press	5	10,8,6,4,2
barbell curls	4	12,10,8,6
skull crushers	5	12,10,8,6,2
hammer curls	4	12,10,8,6
barbell triceps curls	4	12,10,8,6
lunges	4	10,8,8,6

Weeks 3 and 4

Days 1 and 3

exercise	sets	reps
barbell bench press	5	8,6,4,2,1
close-grip lat pull downs	4	8,8,8,8
barbell military press	5	8,6,4,2,1
leg curls	5	10,8,6,4,2
good mornings	4	15,15,15,15
incline barbell bench press	5	8,6,4,2,1
seated cable rows	4	8,8,8,8

Days 2 and 4

exercise	sets	reps
squats	5	10,8,6,4,2
dead lift	5	10,8,6,4,2
preacher curls	4	12,10,8,6
triceps push downs	4	12,10,8,6
reverse curls	4	12,10,8,6
barbell triceps curls	4	12,10,8,6
standing calf raises	4	20,20,20,20

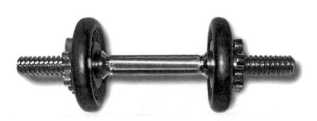

Program Level V
Strength Training
Two-Day Split 4 days per week
Upper & lower body training on different days

Weeks 1 and 2

Days 1 and 3

exercise	sets	reps
barbell bench press	5	8,6,4,2,1
wide-grip lat pull downs	4	8,8,8,8
barbell military press	5	8,6,4,2,1
hammer curls	4	12,10,8,6
close-grip barbell bench press	4	10,10,8,8
bent-over barbell rows	4	8,8,8,8
incline barbell bench press	5	8,6,4,2,1

Days 2 and 4

exercise	sets	reps
squats	5	10,8,6,4,2
leg press	5	10,8,6,4,2
standing calf raises	4	20,20,20,20
lunges	4	10,8,8,6
leg extensions	4	8,8,6,6
leg curls	4	8,8,6,6
dead lift	4	8,6,4,2
seated calf raises	4	20,20,20,20

Weeks 3 and 4

Days 1 and 3

exercise	sets	reps
barbell bench press	5	8,6,4,2,1
close-grip lat pull downs	4	8,8,8,8
barbell military press	5	8,6,4,2,1
reverse curls	4	12,10,8,6
incline barbell bench press	4	10,10,8,8
T-bar rows	4	8,8,8,8
barbell triceps curls	5	12,10,8,6,2

Days 2 and 4

exercise	sets	reps
leg press	5	10,8,6,4,2
squats	5	10,8,6,4,2
lunges	4	10,8,6,4,2
dead lift	4	10,8,8,6
leg curls	4	8,8,6,6
leg extensions	4	8,8,6,6
standing calf raises	4	8,6,4,2

Program Level V
Strength Training
Two-Day Split 4 days per week
Upper & lower body training on the same day
Synergistic Training

Weeks 1 and 2

Days 1 and 3

exercise	sets	reps
barbell bench press	5	8,6,4,2,1
barbell military press	5	8,6,4,2,1
incline barbell bench press	5	8,6,4,2,1
leg curls	5	10,8,6,4,2
close-grip barbell bench press	4	10,10,8,8
good mornings	4	15,15,15,15
skull crushers	5	12,10,8,6,2

Days 2 and 4

exercise	sets	reps
wide-grip lat pull downs	4	8,8,8,8
hammer curls	4	12,10,8,6
squats	5	10,8,6,4,2
leg extensions	4	8,8,6,6
bent-over barbell rows	4	8,8,8,8
lunges	4	10,8,8,6
T-bar rows	4	8,8,8,8

Weeks 3 and 4

Days 1 and 3

exercise	sets	reps
barbell bench press	5	8,6,4,2,1
barbell military press	5	8,6,4,2,1
incline barbell bench press	5	8,6,4,2,1
leg curls	5	10,8,6,4,2
barbell triceps curls	4	10,10,8,8
standing calf raises	4	20,20,20,20
triceps pull downs	4	12,10,8,6

Days 2 and 4

exercise	sets	reps
close-grip lat pull downs	4	8,8,8,8
reverse curls	4	12,10,8,6
leg press	5	10,8,6,4,2
leg extensions	4	8,8,6,6
bent-over barbell rows	4	8,8,8,8
dead lift	5	10,8,6,4,2
seated cable rows	4	8,8,8,8

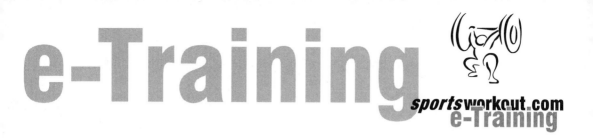

e-Training

sportsworkout.com
e-Training

Would you become **a better athlete** with your very own sport-specific strength and conditioning coach at your fingertips, **24 hours a day?**

All of these services can normally be purchased for well **over $400**. And usually, that's just for a general personal trainer. Now you can take your skills to the next level with your very own **sports trainer.**

Let our team of experts help you train specifically for your sport and we guarantee your athletic performance improves.

➤ **Customized Program Development** *($90 value!)* We will customize a workout program designed specifically for YOU.

➤ **Unlimited, in-depth responses** to all your sport-specific training questions *(normally $110 an hour!*

➤ **Track all of your results** with our customized "e-Charts", and see your improvements on paper.

Get your own personal sport-specific trainer now at
www.SportsWorkout.com or call **1-866-SWORKOUT (796-7568)**

Membership

sportsworkout.com
Membership

SportsWorkout.com

introduces Ryan Lee's Sport-Specific membership, the world's largest strength & conditioning online membership site!

Even the best in the business agree this membership is invaluable:

"Simply the best and most complete sports training resource I've ever used. If you are serious about improving your sports performance, I highly recommend joining today!"

Duane Carlisle
NFL Philadelphia Eagles Speed Consultant

"I was just introduced to your site by a colleague of mine and I wanted to let you know how impressed I was. I will certainly recommend that my athletes check out your site."

Matt Nichol
NHL Toronto Maple Leafs Head Strength Coach

6 months of access to:

➡ Over 5,000 pages of sport-specific articles, programs, and training tips created by professional strength coaches

➡ FREE UNLIMITED Sports Training Consulting via email with a detailed response guaranteed within 48 hours ($900 monthly value!)

➡ Members Only discussion forum with some of the brightest minds in sports training

➡ New articles, programs, video clips, & exercise images added every week

➡ Audio interviews with professional strength coaches

Bonus Items!

➡ The Ultimate Guide to Weight Training for Sports ($37 value!)

➡ Fitness Training e-Charts ($15 value!)

Free Shipping & Handling!

If you order now, we'll pay all shipping costs, and have all bonus items delivered to your door absolutely free!

All for just **$67**! And for a very limited time, if you join today you will also receive an **extra 6 months** added to your membership, **completely free**!

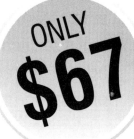

ONLY $67

Get **$5** off with Promo Code 9942

Go to **www.SportsWorkout.com** or call **1-866-SWORKOUT (796-7568)** to Ord